Praise for *A Better Death*

'Death is a subject most of us try to avoid, and all of us need to discuss. I can't imagine a better starting point for that conversation than Ranjana Srivastava's illuminating, inspiring and intensely practical book. The things we most want in a doctor – kindness, compassion, empathy and the reassuring blend of technical skill and professional integrity – are all here, shining through every word'
Hugh Mackay AO, author of *The Good Life*

'A book brimming with pathos and profound insights on facing death with compassion, kindness and forgiveness, for ourselves and those we may be caring for who are dying. In helping us grapple with our own mortality, with unflinching honesty and pragmatism, Dr Srivastava empowers us to live our lives to the full with an urgency and authenticity that will transform all our lives for the better'
Kon Karapanagiotidis OAM, author of
The Power of Hope

'At last, a book to help us prepare for the end of life. With tremendous warmth and wisdom, Dr Srivastava is a compassionate guide – there is comfort here, but also practical advice about the issues we will all face, and how to die with kindness, courage and perhaps, if we are lucky, grace'
Caroline Baum, author of *Only*

'Equal parts moving and informative, this book will leave an indelible mark on anyone looking to cultivate meaning and purpose in life' *Australian Women's Weekly*

'Ranjana Srivastava is the wisest of doctors. *A Better Death* brings together a wealth of experience both as an oncologist and as a human being. Srivastava knows that death is far more than a clinical problem. It is the end point of a complex journey, and medicine is only one of the resources that the traveller might require. This book is alive to all the other needs such as friendship, honesty, purpose, touch, love and gratitude. Even a cup of tea. Dr Srivastava shares many stories from her work and does so in an uplifting and forthright manner. *A Better Death* exudes a calm and positive energy from every page. It is the perfect balm for a fearful and technocratic world. It celebrates the mystery of life'
Michael McGirr, author of *Books that Saved My Life*

'Doctor Srivastava takes your hand in these pages, and leads you skilfully but gently along the road to the end of life. She lights that way vividly and with great thoroughness, as she knows it well, both by heart and by practice. You may be reluctant, but Dr Srivastava is irresistibly convincing and wise. Few among us will have the privilege of Dr Srivastava by our side, but this book is surely the next best thing'
Morag Zwartz, author of *Being Sam*

'With her distinctive combination of empathy and vision, Dr Ranjana Srivastava has written an indispensable book full of warm and wise advice on how to care for those we love at the end of their lives. Further, she invites each of us to consider how we live now, and to think about our own mortality with a new and clear-eyed compassion. What a gift! Read it and give it to everyone you love'
Kate Richards, author of *Madness: A Memoir*

A better death

Also by Dr Ranjana Srivastava

What It Takes to Be a Doctor

A Cancer Companion: An oncologist's advice on diagnosis, treatment and recovery

After Cancer: A guide to living well

So It's Cancer: Now What? An expert's guide to what you need to know

Dying for a Chat: The communication breakdown between doctors and patients

Tell Me the Truth: Conversations with my patients about life and death

A better death

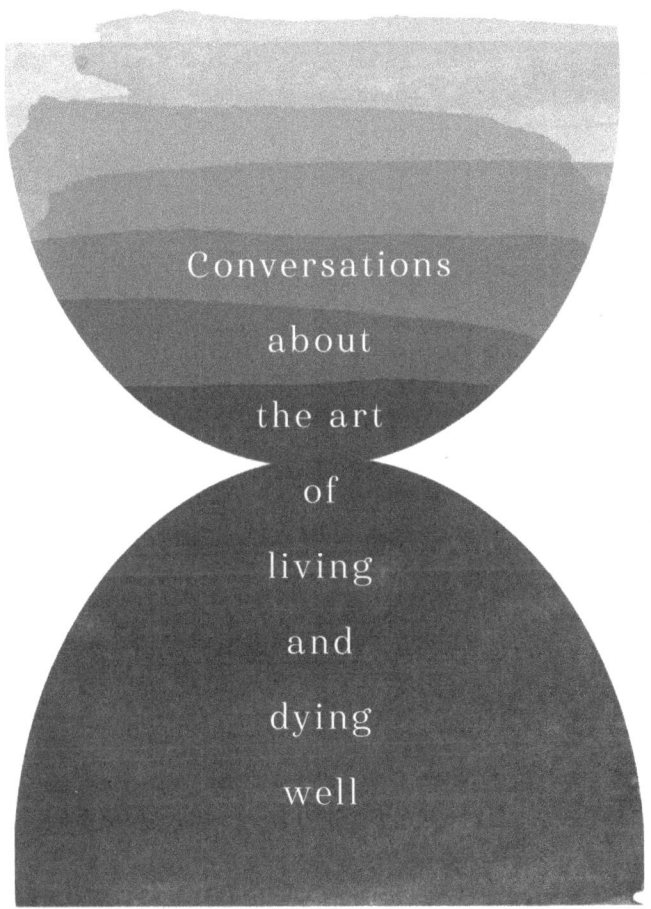

Conversations about the art of living and dying well

Dr Ranjana Srivastava

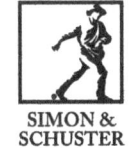

SIMON & SCHUSTER

London · New York · Sydney · Toronto · New Delhi

A CBS COMPANY

A BETTER DEATH: CONVERSATIONS ABOUT THE ART OF LIVING AND
DYING WELL
First published in Australia in 2019 by
Simon & Schuster (Australia) Pty Limited
Suite 19A, Level 1, Building C, 450 Miller Street, Cammeray, NSW 2062

10 9 8 7 6 5 4 3

A CBS Company
Sydney New York London Toronto New Delhi
Visit our website at www.simonandschuster.com.au

© Ranjana Srivastava 2019

All rights reserved. No part of this publication may be reproduced, stored in a retrieval system, or transmitted in any form or by any means, electronic, mechanical, photocopying, recording or otherwise, without prior permission of the publisher.

 A catalogue record for this book is available from the National Library of Australia

Cover design and illustration by Lisa White
Typeset by Midland Typesetters, Australia
Printed and bound in Australia by Griffin Press

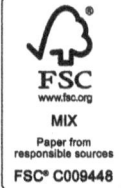 The paper this book is printed on is certified against the Forest Stewardship Council® Standards. Griffin Press holds FSC chain of custody certification SGS-COC-005088. FSC promotes environmentally responsible, socially beneficial and economically viable management of the world's forests.

Ars longa, vita brevis
The art is long, life short.

Hippocrates

For my patients, who teach me

Contents

What I have learnt about dying well	xv
A day in the life	xxv
Part 1 The values of those who die well	1
Believing	5
Acceptance	15
Meaning	27
Forgiveness	39
Equanimity	47
Kindness	59
Gratitude	69
Part 2 Conversations	79
What doctors say, what patients hear	85
Giving patients the worst news	91
How people die	103
Deciding where to die	113
Getting the best care at the end of life	125
Letting go	133

Part 3 Advice for patients and their families	141
Handling conflict within families	147
Friendship and grief	157
Deciding between work and rest	167
Caring for a loved one with dementia	175
Helping our loved ones die comfortably	183
Being a good advocate for the dying	193
Ensuring the whole family gets help	201
Planning ahead	209
The pros and cons of clinical trials	217
Protecting our health	229
Tackling pain at the end of life	237
What to do about denial	245
Dealing with a sudden death	255
Facing the aftermath	269
Epilogue	283
Acknowledgements	287
About the Author	291

A better death

What I have learnt about dying well

I ENTERED MEDICAL SCHOOL with stars in my eyes. After all, doesn't everyone? Crossing the threshold of the cavernous lecture theatre for the first time, I dreamt of changing the world. The portraits of eminent clinicians that lined the corridors never seemed to me as distant things to be admired; rather, they were a living inspiration to earn the privilege of being a doctor.

Like so many young doctors, I was uncertain about my future. I met brilliant physicians and skilled surgeons who excelled in one area, but I always wondered whose job it was to embrace the whole of the patient, especially when things went downhill. Many times, I saw a laser-like focus on the disease dissipate to nothingness when the treatment failed. This happened especially when people were dying. It was often unintentional, but when a specialist slowly detached from dying patients and their families at a time when they most needed help to navigate what came next, it was really a form of abandonment. Consequently, the people who inspired me were those who chose to stay with patients to the end, who saw their duty in larger terms. They recognised that the end of treatment did not mean the end of care. They were good doctors but importantly, they were thoughtful people and I was moved by what powerful consolation they had to offer.

Since the earliest stages of my career, I was struck by how lonely the end of life could be. I met helpless patients and their loved ones who didn't know what to expect at the end of life. I noticed the strain of carers who bickered with each other and fought against their internal conflicts. But I also breathed the calm of patients who had made peace with dying and sensed the quiet determination of relatives joined by common purpose. I admiringly watched social workers deal with practical matters like paying off debts and recording a legacy and then finding time for existential questions that didn't have straightforward answers but nonetheless deserved attention: Why me? Why now?

I shouldn't have been surprised that one sentiment I repeatedly encountered was how much patients valued the

Dr Ranjana Srivastava

kindness of their doctors. Dying patients and their relatives obviously appreciated the advocacy of their doctors in keeping them well but they reserved their most profound gratitude for those who cared for them and about them at the end of life.

The other crucial thing I learnt was how ill-equipped medicine is to help patients deal with the universal fact of life that is their death. Patients and caregivers described how difficult it was to get to the truth of an illness and how unprepared they felt to make major decisions about how far to go and what to do. For every patient who dismissed the need to talk about death and dying, there were many more who needed help to say the things they meant to say and do the things they longed to do.

Six years of medical school. Twelve more years of training. Eventually, I followed in the footsteps of a mentor to become a specialist in two areas: oncology and internal medicine.

Oncologists specialise in the diagnosis and management of cancer and possess detailed knowledge about cancer treatments, their relative merits, and their side effects.

Internal medicine physicians care for a broad range of patients such as those who have heart disease, stroke, diabetes, dementia, infections, chronic pain, lung disease and other chronic medical conditions. Nine out of ten people over the age of 65 have at least one common chronic condition and many patients consult a specialist for each organ. The most important role of an internal medicine physician is to avoid piecemeal medicine and provide a cohesive approach to the whole person.

My main work is as an oncologist. For three months each year, I also work as an internal medicine specialist. For two decades, I have worked in a public hospital located in one of the country's most multicultural and also most socioeconomically depressed regions – an area of high crime, entrenched poverty and crippling illiteracy. Practising medicine in this environment and effecting change is twice as hard. I have felt despondent, been threatened and robbed, yet I have never thought to leave. Because tucked away amongst these oppressive problems is something else: an unparalleled chance to learn not only the vagaries of medicine but importantly, how people from different corners of the world experience life and face death.

My patients hail from a staggering 160 different countries. Many don't speak English as a first language, follow different faiths and have unique customs and traditions. In this melting pot, I care for professionals and labourers, migrants and asylum seekers, people blessed with friends and those who have no one, those who've made it in life and those who doubt they ever will. I consult priests and chaplains, imams, monks and rabbis who come to tend dying patients. I observe who keeps vigil at the bedside, what binds a grieving family, and how different people learn to let go, and I realise that this is in fact the unprecedented and richest reward of my work – a chance to contemplate a meaningful life and a peaceful death.

As an oncologist, I see how death from cancer is often emotional and public. Many professionals are dedicated to caring for terminally ill cancer patients who are the beneficiaries of enthusiastic healthcare funding, community sympathy and a steadily increasing pool of resources. It should be so. Unfortunately, in the role of an internal medicine specialist, I see that the same can't be said of patients dying from dementia, heart disease, stroke, infection, or progressive organ failure. Their death is often slow, their trajectory unpredictable and their dying no less tragic, but such patients and their family members frequently find themselves short of information and counsel at a vulnerable time.

Needless to say, it's not only the elderly who die; people in their thirties and forties also die of terminal illness, usually with an entirely different set of needs, regrets and responsibilities. A just and humane society recognises that all of us deserve to die well.

We all desire basic independence and dignity; where there is suffering, many of us think it's preferable to see a life end than turn into a series of slow disasters. Modern medicine has made this an all-too-familiar sight but even when such patients die our relief is tinged with sadness for what the death represents:

the loss of a unique individual as well as a beloved partner, a devoted parent, a loved child, or a fond sibling.

Being a doctor has taught me that discoveries, treatments and cures are important and exciting but what's even more important is the ability of doctors to help patients navigate what happens when the discoveries disappoint, treatments fail, and cures never arrive. Somehow, amid all the advances of drugs and technology, medicine forgot to allow for people to die. Academic journals, scientific gatherings and popular media are rife with stories about the next big breakthrough in medicine, some of which are a just cause for celebration. But we are all mortal and each one of us must contend with the great subject of our own dying. This is where medicine often falls silent, losing its confident tread, ambivalent about how exactly to mention the obvious: that we are all slowly dying and that being afraid of death or not talking about it isn't going to make it go away.

Doctors play an instrumental role in end-of-life care. They can ease pain and bring peace by helping people understand that it's time to call a halt to futile and uncomfortable treatment and ponder some bigger questions.

I experienced this myself at a young age when my first pregnancy suddenly ended in the late-term loss of both twins. In the course of a single day, I went from a completely fit woman and a newly-minted oncologist to a terrified patient who was losing both twins through a rare condition I had never even heard of. The bad news was piling up too fast for my shaken mind to absorb it all. But amidst the confusion, I asked the veteran obstetrician a single question that would be my saving grace: 'Will the twins die?'

To his eternal credit, and my infinite gratitude, he responded yes. Then, he quietly and patiently described why. His eyes were moist and his sympathy palpable.

I can't overestimate the significance of this straight answer that removed my doubt, stopped my husband and I from looking for answers, and set us on the path to acceptance. The death of the twins was always inevitable; but our experience could have been tainted in so many ways. The right words spoken by the doctor at the right time not only made the sorrow bearable but also put calm and courage in our next steps. The twins were laid to rest and we went on to have three healthy children.

For a doctor who started out dreaming of making change, it's taken nearly two decades of practice, searing personal loss and soul-searching along the way to realise that a fine medical education and costly training can be justifiably used for a purpose other than extending the lives of patients – doctors can also help patients die well.

After all, some day we'll all find ourselves in the situation of caring for a loved one or, perhaps more importantly, caring for ourselves at the end of life. None of us on our own could expect to gain all the practicality, knowledge and wisdom needed to die well, but we can all learn something from sharing stories. As the philosopher Michel de Montaigne said, it is good to rub and polish our brain against that of others.

The *Mahabharata* is a three-thousand-year-old major Indian epic that holds sage lessons for the modern era. It contains a dialogue between a celestial figure and a nobleman. 'What is the most surprising thing in the world?' the spirit asks Yudhishthira.

He responds: 'Day after day man sees countless people die but still, he acts and thinks as if he will live forever.'

This is at once a profound philosophical question for humanity and a personal quest for every human being.

I KNOW THAT MY PATIENTS would be delighted, humbled and ever so proud that they could illuminate the lives of others. Indeed, there is a lot to learn from the experiences of people dying in this extraordinary time of progress. Many of my patients wish they had more time left for family and better friendships, more laughter, less conflict, more contentment, less stress. But with support and advocacy, they also come to recognise that amid all the twists and turns, there are many moments of happiness, fulfilment and discovery to be cherished that give meaning to life, no matter what its duration. This knowledge and its accompanying consolations can be found if we look for them. The power to achieve a better death lies within each of us.

My greatest hope for this book is that it gives a sense of control to readers. Popular culture might frame it so but dying is not about accepting defeat or letting go. Death is a universal destiny, not the price we pay for living; rather, a natural conclusion of living. Dying well is about treating ourselves and others in the last act of life with grace and goodwill. We can persist with qualities that exacerbate our suffering or adopt those that celebrate the time we have left. For the bereaved, death need not be associated with intractable grief but spur the creation of a hopeful legacy. This is why, for all of us, a better death should not be a mere hope but a worthy goal that honours the life we have led.

A day in the life

'How do you keep calm when you see such terrible things?' my host quizzed me at a social event. I felt relieved, yet vaguely guilty that the tumult in my mind was not apparent on my face.

Today was gut-wrenchingly difficult, I wanted to tell her. The seven years spent in the shadow of a cancer diagnosis had been broadly kind to my patient, Lucy, although I could appreciate that at age forty-five she might not concur with my definition of kindness, which considered her improved prognosis, a lack of hospitalisation, stable scans and her ability to continue working as a beautician.

Also, her medications hadn't caused unacceptable side

effects; she had avoided regular blood tests; and she was not beholden to her doctors to tell her when to take a holiday.

What this definition did not acknowledge, however, is that she had an incurable malignancy which would one day result in her untimely death, and Lucy felt considerable pressure to make each year, even each month, count as if it were her last. Every annual event such as a school concert, dance performance, or Christmas contained the poignancy of it potentially being her last. No one knew. But a silent clock was ticking somewhere and there was all that living to do before it ran out.

Her medications were not toxic, but they were by no means benign, and she had to bend her mind to get used to them. The catalogue of irritations including insomnia, aches and pains, diminished libido, fatigue and a vague but permanent dread might seem mild or expected according to the drug insert; for Lucy, they were the necessary price for staying alive. Medicine could not restore her former self; life was about adjusting to change. It was an important distinction: every time I assure a patient that a new drug isn't 'too toxic', what I'm really telling them is that on the whole, the trade-off is good but there will be days when it won't be so. A new uncertainty has entered their life that medicine will not be able to displace.

However, doctors must still be able to relate to the illness of their patients.

Dr Ranjana Srivastava

'I feel fine,' Lucy sometimes reported with puzzlement as I frowned over some test abnormality.

'I'm so pleased. Remember, not all cancers cause problems.'

What I omitted was to say, 'But one day, you and I will both feel devastated.'

'Will it ever go away?'

'Not completely.'

Sometimes succinct answers are both necessary and useful. They can feel cruel, but they are also my insurance: when a patient says, 'I had no idea', I know that isn't completely true.

However, in Lucy's case numerous such exchanges over the years had lulled us into a sense of security, which no one questioned as being inevitably temporary. The beneficiary was a wife and mother who welcomed the reprieve granted her at every visit. Why begrudge her the time in which she had seen her children grow? Why cloud their holidays with dire predictions? She was the good news story no one wanted to end.

I had told her that she didn't need scans at her most recent visit, but her family doctor arranged them to be helpful. Now, Lucy handed over the films and I silently lined up the images, having learnt long ago how much patients disliked small talk during this ritual. I fleetingly wished I'd had prior notice of the scans, but Lucy looked so well that I assumed there was nothing to find.

A day in the life

Suddenly, my heart quickened at the sight of unexpected new disease staring back at me. Blinking my eyes and peering more closely didn't change that. The changes were small, but definitely present and involved a vital organ, her liver. They were a harbinger of the troubles that lay ahead, the troubles that we'd pushed to the back of our mind for so many years.

The first news of disease progression is devastating for doctors and patients. The floor shifted under me.

'All good, doctor?' Her tone was typically soft and respectful.

Many times, in the past, I had turned back to face her with a reassuring smile and a vigorous nod, a sign that things were stable. But in the split second before I turned around this time, I knew that I held the knowledge that would irretrievably change her life. From here on, things would never be the same. Gone were the relaxed appointments and the easy banter about family life and school holidays; in their place a revolving door of fears and concerns. A literal pronouncement that her cancer had spread would shatter her hopes and convince her that she was imminently dying. Bland advice that there wasn't much to say would be deceptive. I tensed with the task of arranging my words and expression with extra care.

I sat down so Lucy and I were eye to eye.

'Actually, there are some new changes in the liver,' I began, with a calm I didn't feel. Her usually amiable expression faded as I continued, 'They represent cancer.' This felt like a needless assault, but it was even more unbearable when patients sighed, 'Thank god they're only spots.' Every oncologist learns this the hard way. 'I know this is disappointing but it's very small progression and there are many promising drugs.'

I stopped there, knowing the rest would go unheard. At the inevitable progression of their cancer, some patients weep, others are bewildered and yet others slam the desk in anger. She sat absolutely still and, much as I yearned to stifle the silence with my own noisy plans, I took my cue from her. My silence was an appropriate homage to a lull that would never return.

Her face crumpled with disappointment, she asked to see her scans and I pointed out the silent invaders. She asked if she must start the new drug today and I said no. She asked if, despite my disappointment, I would still be her doctor and at this, my reserve crumbled.

'I'm not disappointed in you,' I protested, tears now stinging the back of my eyes. 'I'm just sorry it came back.'

Her phone rang, and she said apologetically, 'That's my mum, she always checks in.'

Lucy's mother attended the appointments her husband couldn't, so she'd never be alone. Today, Lucy had felt so well that she'd come by herself. This was a tight-knit family and I hated to imagine the ripple effect of my pronouncement. I made myself think of the fact that the children had strong supports beyond their mother.

'My mind feels wobbly,' she said softly. I knew why. Inside, she was already thinking a thousand things – whether she had taken her medication faithfully for all those years, what about that weekend she forgot, if that pain she suffered last month was a sign, what would she tell her mother, what if the new drug didn't work, how would the children react, how much should she tell them, would she grow suddenly unwell now, would there be time to finish remaining things?

I imagine I'd be the same and there seemed to be nothing remotely comforting to say, so I told her what I thought. 'I will look after you to the best of my ability.'

If Lucy was unsettled, she didn't show it outwardly, instead leaving the room politely and leaving me with my thoughts.

Did she sink into her car seat and cry or did she plug her emotions to drive straight home? Did she call her mum back or temporarily spare her the sorrow? Did her husband take the day off or save up precious sick leave? And what did she do that night – feign normality at the dinner table or tell her children the truth? That afternoon, as I calculated the dose of her next chemotherapy, striving to give her all the benefit minus the worst side effects, I was also thinking of the countless calculations she would inflict on herself about how long she had left to live.

I couldn't help worrying if she'd lost a little faith in me because I didn't order the scan. Did she consider me blasé about her illness? Did she fear that I'd let her down again? I tried not to let these worries discompose me, remembering that they're common to doctors whose work knits close bonds with their patients.

After she left, I saw other patients. Some were straightforward; others needed encouragement. Some were experiencing hiccups in their treatment and required interventions, from minor troubleshooting to a perhaps unexpected conversation about a poor prognosis. Every patient needed attention, kindness and, occasionally, a curtailing of my impatience.

But in a corner of my mind, I kept thinking that I couldn't leave any stone unturned for Lucy. So, I vexed over drugs, trials and the literature. In between, I dreaded meeting her elderly mother and shuddered at the thought of spotting her children in the waiting room. My mind would run ahead of itself and picture her in hospice. I'd hastily rewind it and imagine still undiscovered drugs keeping her well indefinitely. And even as all these sentiments jostled for attention, I reminded myself that I'd been here before and would be here again. These occurrences are an oncologist's burden and privilege. It's why some doctors say they could never do this job – and others can't imagine doing anything else.

I kept thinking of how Monday mornings are the hardest, in spite of the fact that I've never considered my work a chore. The respite of a weekend is erased the moment I walk into the ward to meet patients admitted to hospital over the weekend. Monday morning brings me face to face with patients whose anxieties have swelled over an entire weekend and who are convinced that they are in the worst possible situation. Some are right – people know enough to avoid coming to hospital on the weekend unless they are seriously unwell – but many have smaller problems that can be treated with antibiotics, painkillers or plain reassurance.

Unlike the patients I see in my clinic, many of the ward patients are new to me. I might later inherit their care or learn they already have an oncologist at a different hospital. Other doctors might have promised them that come Monday everything will be clearer but often it just isn't so. Good medicine takes time, though the labyrinthine hospital system can drown even the most capable patients in a sea of vulnerability.

On the rounds, my team gives news of improvement, deterioration and, occasionally, impending death. I often rue that there is no chance for us to ease into work – one of my routine tasks on Mondays is to tell total strangers that I'm an oncologist and they have cancer. There is no ideal time for it but starting the week like this is to rush headlong into emotions that got parked for the weekend. It's also a powerful reminder of the necessity of treating life with respect and people with consideration.

Dr Ranjana Srivastava

The stories of my patients are confronting at first sight. A common theme is a lack of acceptance of death as a corollary of life. In fact, tackling this hurdle uses up most of my time. There are many reasons for this: the reticence of doctors and the reluctance of patients to discuss dying and the attitude in modern society that every problem has an instant solution and every ailment a quick fix.

Denial of death is so common that many of my consultations with the sickest patients hinge on broaching the notion that we are all mortal. Interns and junior doctors may never have heard such a conversation. I prepare them by insisting that we can entertain other things – the latest blockbuster therapy, the miracle cure on the evening news, the neighbour whose disease simply vanished – but we must never forget to bring our patients back to the truth: that we have limited lives and it is for us to decide how best to spend our time. This, I believe, is the hardest part of all medicine.

The belief that a conversation is needed doesn't make it easier to have. If it were so, all the great lectures, compelling stories and grassroots movements about dying well would have worked by now. Ordering another test or prescribing a last-ditch drug requires the mere tap of a keyboard; a conversation about something as significant as mortality takes space and time – and hence money – and there's always the risk of alienating a patient. No one objects to the doctor who orders an extra test; complaints abound about those who declare there is no treatment left to give.

Patients are willing to put up with a lot but the longer I've been a doctor the more I realise that to be a doctor is to care about much more than organs and drugs. Indeed, the burst of information technology has set unprecedented amounts of scientific literature, research and innovation at our feet, more than any doctor can possibly grapple with. Where there is more and more data, there seems less and less heart, but what has never changed is the requirement for a doctor to approach the human condition with a gentle touch.

Especially when it comes to dying, what we ask of our doctors isn't just professional confidence but also kindness, comfort and consolation. We long to meet someone who has mulled over the idea of mortality and understands what it is like to be cloaked in a set of desires, fears and hopes. We want to be cared for by someone who will take the time to listen to us, advise us but ultimately empower us to make our own decisions. Patients are best served by such doctors – and it's the duty of all of medicine to aspire to this ambitious but by no means impossible task.

My most onerous responsibility as a doctor is helping my patients come to terms with dying. Who knows, I ponder, one day I might be like them – plaintive and puzzled, inwardly fearful that I might be dying but not daring to think any further because of the sheer thought, work and heartache involved. Our mortality is guaranteed but, sadly, conversations about dying aren't. In fact, in an era of unprecedented medical progress where interventions can easily spill into futile medical care which is individually painful and societally wasteful, it's never been more important to think about how we want to die. But if we treat the subject of death as insurmountable, we risk depriving ourselves of a considered life and a peaceful death. We're born with many instincts and reflexes, but we have to develop the ones that tell us how to live and die well. That's okay, because we humans have a great capacity to learn from others.

The final consult of the day was with the son of a patient, who burst into tears as he handed me an envelope. 'I promised myself I wouldn't cry, but then I saw you.'

'That's my job,' I shrugged, half-despondently, making him laugh.

His card thanked me for a curious thing: 'for worrying about Dad, but not always in front of him'. It applauded my whole team for 'showing compassion even when we all knew you couldn't save him'. It wouldn't have struck me to do otherwise, but his words were like raindrops to parched earth. I knew how much the writer's elderly father had wanted to keep on living – sometimes, we measure the strength of a doctor–patient relationship by a patient's longevity but that's unfair to everyone. Trust, empathy and communication rank highly too. When dealing with the challenges of the dying, the antidote to our own vulnerability lies in discovering meaningful ways to help them.

Knowing ourselves is a very good start, but to die well, we must articulate our thoughts and make purposeful decisions towards achieving a better death. This has never been more important: I've lost count of the patients and families who are plunged into needless grief because they're unable to navigate increasingly complex healthcare systems that have an impetus to push for more when less might be better.

Our ancestors were acutely aware of the ubiquity of death. Babies died; women succumbed to childbirth; infections, poverty, starvation and accidents wantonly destroyed lives.

'Death is as sure for that which is born as birth for that which is dead. Therefore, grieve not for what is inevitable,' exhorts the *Bhagavad Gita*, an ancient Hindu text.

'Let us eat and drink because tomorrow we die,' counsels the Book of Isaiah in the Old Testament.

On a humbler note, I grew up listening to my elderly Indian relatives talk openly about a time they wouldn't live to see. There was no discernible judgment, desire or angst in their voices – they talked about death as we might about sunrise or the ocean tides, each with an inevitability of its own.

Unlike past eras, death in modern times is rarely sudden or

unexpected. We're living longer, healthier lives and, compared to past generations when it was quite common to lose a parent or a grandparent at a young age, many generations can now expect to grow old together. Few things bring my oldest patients more pride than counting the number of grandchildren and great-grandchildren in their lives. Their elders would have been lucky to see their own child grow up.

Today, infection control, better housing and sanitation, improved literacy, prevention programs, and advances in medical technology have made it possible for us to forget about death. We think we'll deal with it another time – next month or next year, when we've negotiated retirement, when the youngest child has left home, or when something actually goes wrong. After all, the world's full of people who are alive, isn't it?

Alas, in doing so, we fail to invest our lives with the thought and meaning they deserve before circumstances force us into this reckoning. I see this frequently when I talk to patients about their limited life expectancy and ask what's important to them in their remaining days. They look at me with confusion and reply with utter sincerity, 'I don't know; I never thought this would happen to me.'

In death, I've seen awe-inspiring courage, indescribable love, remarkable sacrifice, insurmountable anger and genuine bewilderment. A good death can be hard to define because it means different things to different people, but most of us have an intuitive sense of it when we see it. And while all death stings, there is great consolation to be found in a peaceful death, while its opposite can leave long-lasting lament and soul-searching.

'Even death is not to be feared by those who have lived wisely', Lord Buddha said. The conversations, prayers and meditations of our elders contained many reminders of our mortality and the importance of leading a simple and meaningful life. Global progress has gradually led us away from such active considerations, making our lives fast and far-flung and our relationships transactional. The thrilling march of medicine has tamed diseases once thought incurable and brought both quantity and quality to millions of lives, but in the process has sheltered us from the idea that our lives are ultimately limited. The vast majority of deaths in the western world now take place in an institution, but medical education teaches doctors very little about the twilight of life and end-of-life care.

An important part of being an oncologist is caring about and for people who are dying. Consequently, I've gained a foundation of medical knowledge and practical experience with which to help others navigate death. There may be no joy in tending the dying but there is something else. There is perspective. Doctors who are drawn to my line of work learn about the impermanence of health and the vicissitudes of life. We see how, even inside a failing body, a spirit can still mend, bit by bit. We witness the transformative effect of a loving family. We see how kindness moves mountains like no medicine can. Caring deeply for patients makes us confront our limitations and deal with our own mortal fears. Every day we learn what *really* matters.

Behind me are photographs of my three children, whose happy faces greet me whenever I turn around to find a form. They are beginning to understand what my work entails but mostly, their days are filled with innocence and play as any parent would wish. My children ground me and remind me of my good fortune. But what I find most touching is that the patients just love them. I can't count the number of times their moist eyes have swung from me to the photographs behind me, as if to say, 'If you have children, you must know something about how I feel'. It is at once a formidable and magnificent expectation to rise to.

Modern life is awash with tips on how to live well, reminding us to practise gratitude, meditate, discover meaning and ponder our legacy. Nothing underlines the importance of these things as dwelling on the lives of others and, in turn, our own. For it's not only other people who are dying; we are all dying. To pretend otherwise is naive. But to learn from each other may be the wisest thing we can do with our lives. This is the challenge and consolation that bookends many of my days.

A day in the life

This is not a book I could have contemplated, let alone written, at the beginning of my career. But years of sharing the journey with all kinds of patients with nearly every mentionable illness has equipped me with two beliefs. One, it is possible to die well. Two, doctors owe it to their patients to show them how.

This is not a book that ignores the tremendous and unprecedented advances of science. This is not a book about giving up or giving in. There is a Buddhist proverb that when the student is ready, the master appears. I have found this to be true for some of my most memorable patients, who were leading ordinary lives until they had to contend with their mortality. They didn't have a textbook to help them but plumbed their own depths to decide how to tackle the journey. Similarly, I have met countless carers who would never have imagined being charged with the responsibility of helping a loved one die and hardly thought themselves equal to the task but who rose admirably to the occasion.

And this is the message I want to bring you in this book. I hope this can be a source of inspiration and comfort for one of the most important events of your life.

Dr Ranjana Srivastava

Part 1

The values of those who die well

Our life is what our thoughts make it.
Marcus Aurelius

MARTIN LUTHER, a 16th century theologian, said that in life every man must do two things alone – his own believing and his own dying. Over the years, I've discovered what this really means. People who die well tend to hold certain values and attributes that inform and enrich their whole lives. Compassion, empathy, forgiveness, self-worth, equanimity, acceptance and resilience are all important. We may not have them in equal measure, but we can strive to cultivate them and use them in our interactions.

Amid the turmoil of tackling their illness, my most memorable patients have demonstrated these qualities to ease their own experience and that of those supporting them – their friends and loved ones. They would be proud to know that they left a legacy.

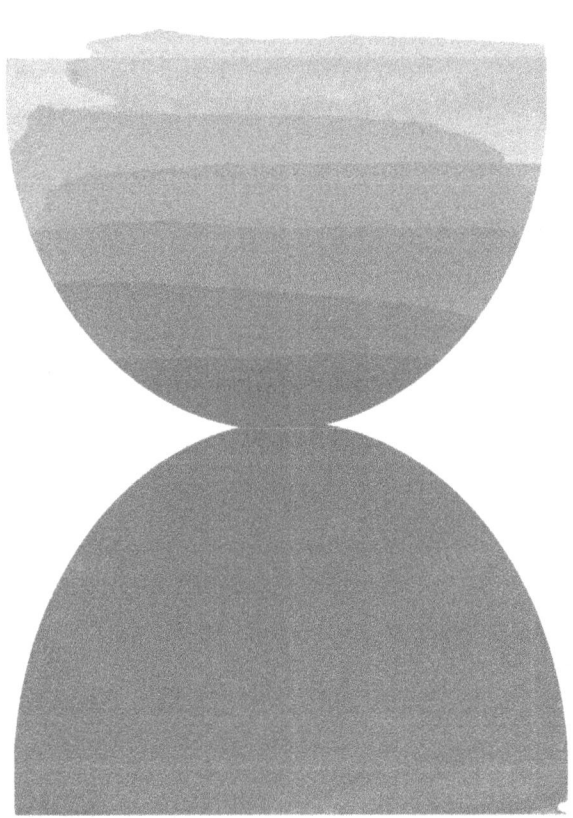

Believing

The most difficult thing in life is to know yourself.
Thales

DYING GIVES RISE TO DEEP EMOTIONS — to sort through and prioritise them is a monumental task that needs genuine attention and quiet space for reflection, planning, mourning, celebration and consolation. But the irony of modern medicine is that amid all that it seeks to do to the *patient*, it doesn't really make room for the *person*.

Simply observing my patients shows me the directions they are impossibly tugged in. Tracking appointments, having tests, ensuring providers communicate, planning transport, finding help, grappling with bills, negotiating work, explaining their illness to others, and avoiding stressful well-wishers — these are just the tasks I hear about, but I imagine the list is never-ending. Indeed, it's reasonable to ask: where's the time for hapless patients to slip out of their exhausting routine and ponder life and legacy?

For a striking number of people, this never happens. I'm amazed by the number of people who say that they have never thought about their death, even in the abstract. Not all of them are young; many are middle-aged and well beyond. But I also regularly meet those who've handled the subject of death admirably in embodiment of the Talmudic quote, 'Live well, it's the greatest revenge.'

Although our death is certain, I imagine we'd rather suspend belief. Every day at work I encounter fixed views that the solution to any illness is but one prescription away and that death can be forestalled by the right idea. The media has a large role to play in this, peppering unrealistic stories with terms like 'game-changer', 'breakthrough' and 'innovative'. Social media compresses them into a format that is digestible but ill-explained. The stories often involve patients who were deemed beyond salvage and laud doctors for rescuing them. Such events are actually rare, but they affect how all of us think about the reach of medicine.

Recently I read a report about a young woman with a rare and aggressive cancer – one most oncologists have never even heard of – who persuaded her doctor to give her a new drug that had not previously been known to work for her disease. She had endured many painful and unsuccessful treatments for years but immediately after taking the new drug, her disease melted away, permitting her to resume work and heavy workouts at the gym.

Although the details were verifiably true, I thought that what matched the patient's remarkable recovery was her oncologist's sanguine observation.

Instead of heralding a miracle, he said he was 'befuddled' by the result, pledging to devote his life to finding out why his patient was an outlier. I wish more doctors would adopt such a balanced approach.

I once met a patient who was expected to die from cancer-related liver failure. Palliative care was called but he refused to talk to anyone who even mentioned end-of-life care. He wanted more chemotherapy, which was unsafe as it could precipitate massive bleeding or a coma, but somehow he twisted an oncologist's arm to prescribe chemotherapy. He died in his chemotherapy chair while receiving treatment, an awful sight for everyone who was present. At the mortality audit, every provider felt contrite and yet everyone knew that it wasn't the first or last time such a thing had occurred.

While dying of cancer is a common fear, the truth is that we are far more likely to be diagnosed with one or more chronic diseases that have no cure and lead to gradual deterioration and death. These diseases include diabetes, cardiovascular disease, chronic kidney failure, lung disease, dementia and mental illness and we tend to underestimate their threat. Nine out of ten Australians over the age of sixty-five have at least one chronic disease and seventy-five per cent of all deaths occur due to a chronic disease. Similar figures exist in many developed countries and developing countries are rapidly catching up with the so-called 'lifestyle' diseases.

To understand why deliberate decision-making in healthcare is more important than ever, it's important to explain the difference between acute and chronic disease.

An acute condition like appendicitis or pneumonia makes people suddenly ill. Here, modern medicine has the capacity to unleash its power and restore health. A painful hernia, a broken bone or a car accident are other examples. When otherwise fit individuals survive these conditions, they can usually put the experience behind them. They don't need to take regular medication or attend long-term check-ups.

Chronic disease behaves differently. As our organs age, they become less resilient and enter a phase of gradual decline. Added insults such as obesity, lack of fitness, smoking and excessive drinking accelerate the decline. Changes to diet and lifestyle can slow the deterioration but not completely reverse it.

Broadly, our quest is to live well and benefit from the discoveries of modern medicine without being held hostage to medical interventions that make life miserable, but this can easily go wrong.

I was recently reminded of this when I met a cognitively impaired man whose wife was distressed about him having dialysis three days each week. By the time he travelled in and out of dialysis, he was exhausted and often confused. He spent the days in between dialysis recovering only to go back to the same situation.

Everyone agreed that he had a poor quality of life but his inability to articulate what he wanted to do when his decade-long renal failure came to a head meant that he entered dialysis by default. His cognition was good enough to make decisions about what to wear or eat but he lacked the capacity to weigh up the consequences of having treatment versus declining it. When there is doubt, medicine frequently errs on the side of overtreatment. Intuitively, no one wants to end up like that man, but the balance between hope and reality is genuinely hard to strike and for people who don't consider their mortality, the task can be next to impossible. This is why in order to live well we have to start believing that we are mortal. This belief is the first step towards making informed decisions at critical times.

One of the great privileges of being an oncologist is seeing how good some people are at this. Amid the turmoil of a life-threatening illness, they somehow make room for calm discussion, acceptance, forgiveness and generosity that eases their own experience of dying and imparts strength to others. We think of them as resilient but, in my view, their resilience is a product of their other attributes. They are resilient because they have a bigger view of life.

As a doctor, I can provide much information to my patients that is backed by evidence and research. Medicine still doesn't have all the answers, but it has more answers than it used to. There are thousands of protocols to manage disease and good advice on how to manage symptoms at the end of life. The fluid world of information makes it easy to obtain a professional opinion via the touch of a keyboard.

But there is no protocol for how to help patients reconcile with their mortality. Here, doctors must listen closely, tread carefully and plumb the depths of their own beliefs. They must interrogate their own conscience, examine their own biases, and decide how much or how little to give a patient.

Doctors don't know how to broach death with their patients because the emphasis of medicine is on sustaining life. Doctors fear death as much as their patients do; perhaps even more because of what they know. And ultimately, doctors humbly recognise that their thoughts on what constitutes a meaningful life and how to die well are just that: no more or less valid than those of the next person.

Dr Ranjana Srivastava

Sometimes I fear that a career in oncology has been prematurely ageing but I hasten to add that it has introduced me to a very satisfying world of patient care. It has also made me engage deeply with what dying well should mean.

First of all, it's hard to contemplate dying without some basic information. Amid the practical things, we should want to know what to expect. Understanding that there are individual variations, what is known about the natural course of our illness? How would aggressive management with its inevitable side effects help in contrast to limited intervention whose aim might be to keep us comfortable? What impact would certain treatments have on the quantity versus quality of life? Some treatments improve both, many don't. We know that many people, especially as they grow older, prioritise independence over prolongation of life. Access to some basic information influences all other important decisions.

The human body is complicated and the process of navigating the healthcare system keeps getting more and more complex. Expert advice is crucial, but one should not be a slave to it, looking to include the counsel of family and friends who have known us as a person first and a patient later. We owe the dying our considered thoughts rather than reflexive responses, which often have to do with chasing miracles. Finally, we should welcome advice from nurses, social workers, allied health professionals and chaplains who usually stay in the background but who can help us live well in ways that are not always apparent to doctors.

More philosophically, we should constantly take stock of the things that bring us pleasure and satisfaction and prioritise them. Most people at the end of life simply don't have the energy to indulge every passion and passing interest. Those who know which pleasures to sacrifice and which to hold on to are often the ones who enjoy the quality of life that proves elusive for so many others. For some of my patients, the ability to read is important. For others, it's living independently, enjoying their garden, or spending time with their children. Recognising what's important to us brings us a step closer to the goal.

We need to know that even the most stoic among us can be ready to die and still be afraid. I commonly encounter such patients on rounds. Some people fear physical experiences like pain, nausea and fatigue. Others are perplexed by emotions like regret, conflict or guilt. Still others find it hard to put a finger on what they are feeling. Seeking help to identify what bothers us and what we can do about it is a sign of maturity.

It isn't easy to contemplate our presence being erased from the world. There's always something else that needs taking care of. Parents want to see their children grow up; the builder wants to complete the house; grandparents want to see another grandchild born. However ordinary we think our lives to be, most of us can find some incentive to keep living.

As onlookers, we must discover sympathy for those who cannot bear to leave the world, but also develop the tools to do better when our time comes. To do justice to the final act of our life, we should want to act with poise and dignity – for ourselves, those we love, and those who love us so deeply that they cannot imagine life without us.

I watch the most profound acts at the end of life and yet I honestly can't say how many I will be able to replicate in my own life. We can't predict whether we will live up to our high expectations, but we should know that, through deliberate thought and conscious action, it is possible to achieve a better death.

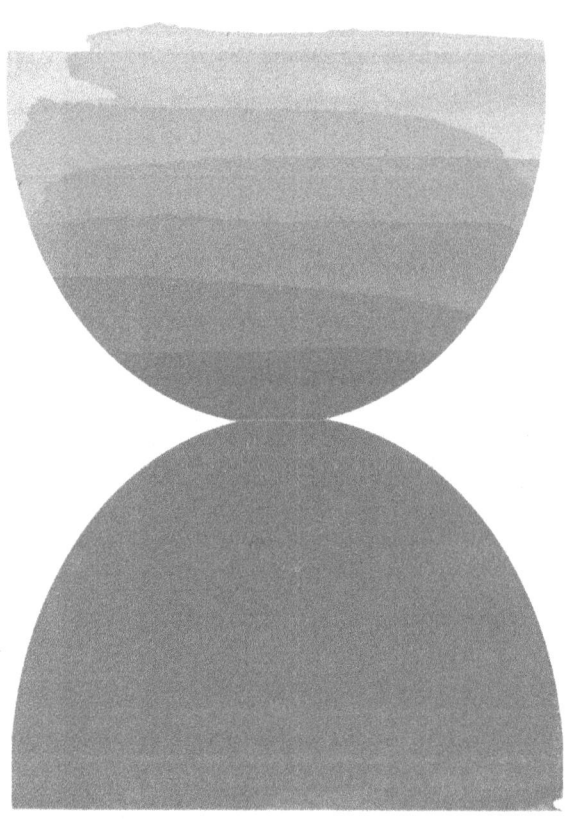

Acceptance

We cannot live better than in seeking to become better.
Socrates

SALLY WAS JUST FORTY when she was diagnosed with advanced cancer. She had four children, the youngest just seven. She'd consulted her doctor to report a persistent stitch in her side after a family holiday, wondering if she'd hiked too vigorously. Instead, the doctor discovered something far more serious.

I wouldn't have met Sally except for her disastrous first experience with another doctor. As anyone who has waited for a medical appointment knows, the process of getting to the actual visit can be quite involved. Initially, Sally saw her GP who agreed with her hunch and prescribed anti-inflammatories. But when the pain didn't subside, Sally had tests that raised the suspicion of cancer. These tests prompted others over the next two weeks and then it was another wait for an appointment with an oncologist.

I can't imagine how heavy those weeks of waiting must have felt, with each result striking a blow, but somehow, Sally and her husband, John, managed to maintain a normal family life while they waited to see what the oncologist would say.

On the day of their appointment, they noted a very busy clinic and waited patiently all afternoon to find out what it meant to have advanced cancer. Afternoon faded into evening and some doctors left. Finally, her name was called out by the only remaining person, a trainee doctor. He looked tired and frazzled and his pager kept beeping. The couple ignored the interruptions and concentrated on the conversation. What happened next would be etched in their memory.

The trainee started by telling Sally outright that she had incurable cancer with a dismal prognosis. However, she could try chemotherapy if she wanted.

'I sat there, completely frozen,' she later told me. 'He behaved like an automaton – there was no sympathy in his voice, no sense of the tragedy we'd been hit with.'

'What does this mean?' John dared to ask, when he found his voice.

What they heard was that Sally needed to start planning to die.

'I laughed at him in disbelief,' Sally recalled. 'I laughed and said, "I have four children. I'll sell my house and everything I own in order to live for them."'

The trainee looked at them tiredly as if he had heard it all before.

Night had fallen by the time Sally and John walked out hand in hand. They had gone to their first oncology appointment with hope, but it had proved too upsetting for words. They had thought they'd be discussing treatment logistics on the way home, but instead they ended up debating how to move to another country to have good treatment. This panic felt so foreign to the usually calm couple that they called a nurse they had briefly met at the hospital to share their consternation. She convinced them to see someone else before deciding. Sally reluctantly agreed, and I had a cancellation, which is how we met.

I have seen many reactions to a cancer diagnosis – patients who are stunned, hyperventilating, sobbing, or occasionally even close to collapse, but what struck me from the minute she walked in was Sally's poise. I knew from reading her history that she had no risk factors for cancer. There was no family history, she herself was young and fit, and had never been in hospital after childbirth. That a stitch in the side turned out to be cancer was bad enough but her experience with the first oncologist had been awful.

Many patients might justifiably start by flagging that experience as a warning to the next doctor, but I'd never have known from Sally's expression that she had met an oncologist the previous day. Her face was wiped clear of any grievance, but when I began with the apology she deserved, her eyes clouded.

'It was late,' she said, peaceably accounting for the unacceptable behaviour. I could see John trying hard to control his emotions.

'I want to forget about that incident and find out everything you know,' Sally continued.

Slowly, I told her the facts. Her cancer was advanced and inoperable. There was nothing she could have done to prevent it and in fact she was part of a growing trend of relatively young people developing cancer. There were treatments to shrink and stabilise her disease. If she benefited from all the available treatments, her life expectancy was between two and three years, and I would do my best to help her get there. My tongue felt stuck at each pronouncement, but I continued because I respected her need to know and understood how important mutual trust was to a therapeutic relationship between us.

Sally and John absorbed the news quietly. I expected her to cry, protest or finally unleash her anger; instead, all she said was, 'Okay, what do I do next?' Much as doctors welcome our job being made easier, I was taken aback by her composed reaction. Patients rarely behaved like this, especially those with a very young family and great responsibility on their shoulders.

My first reaction was to wonder if she had somehow misunderstood the gravity of her situation or was concealing her true feelings but realised that neither seemed the case. People twice her age would be rattled by lesser tragedies, but Sally really did turn out to be the calm, collected woman of my first impressions. And since we were roughly the same age, I took a special interest in her journey that seemed to me like a mother's worst nightmare come alive.

Good news was around the corner. Sally had a great initial response, which buoyed us all. Childlike, I hoped it would last forever, although experience told me otherwise.

When thinking about what the best care means, doctors are taught to ask themselves this 'surprise question' about patients. 'If the patient were to die in the next twelve months, would I be surprised?' The answer is remarkably accurate in predicting survival. While every patient is unique, and every doctor has a different slant on the same facts, this question encourages doctors to think about which interventions are still helping a person with a limited prognosis. With a heavy heart and feeling treacherous, when I applied the surprise question to Sally, I hoped 'Yes' but answered 'No'. There was the potential for far too many things to go wrong.

We all breathed a sigh of relief when the first year passed uneventfully. She fell into a new routine and what she did was determined by how she felt.

Thankfully, Sally mostly stayed well. She took occasional breaks to fit in with school holidays and was able to run a busy household with John. She'd been thinking of returning to work before her illness stopped her. Instead of ruing this, she saw it as an opportunity to devote more time to her children. Much to their delight, she became a helper in the school library and a visible presence in the school canteen. The school community united around her and for a time Sally's life assumed a heartening normality.

I was always intrigued by this normality, which was genuine, but never doubted that it came from a place of great effort. Where many people would have felt dejected, Sally tended to focus on the positive. Yet this never felt like denial; in fact, the opposite; Sally possessed a preternatural sense of acceptance about her fate and knew exactly how she wanted to live her life.

Partway through the second year, things became spitefully difficult. The chemotherapy stopped working and mounting side effects resulted in several hospital visits. Drugs and antibiotics controlled her symptoms but at the expense of making her tired and drowsy. She was honest about her discomfort, but also unflappable. One day, standing by her bed after yet another disturbed night, I realised that my patient was someone with bravery at her core. I concluded that in accepting that she was dying, Sally had seized on a powerful truth: what was happening to her did not define who she was. It was a difficult concept, which she embraced with self-assurance.

This made me recall her early remark that her situation would not alter her core beliefs or her conduct towards others. Consequently, she remained personable and relatable, and in some way, the obvious goodwill this generated must have made her journey more bearable.

One day, conscious of having evoked more sadness, I said feelingly, 'Sally, I'm really sorry you're going through this. I wish there was something I could do.'

Her response stopped me in my tracks.

'But we're all going to die,' she said evenly. 'I guess my time came sooner than usual. You can't help that.'

Instead of being the consoler, I ended up as the consoled. Sally's conduct gave many of us the impetus to match her determination and not be embittered by our fate.

She had always struck me as the engine of the marriage, so I was curious to know how John was coping since all I saw was his valiant but almost wordless support.

'She keeps us all strong,' he said, his voice faltering. He went on to explain how every family member drew inspiration from her. She had told her siblings grieving was okay but helping her with errands was even better. The errands included driving across town to collect a ceramic vase for her mother and ordering fancy dress costumes for her daughters. The siblings rolled their eyes at some of these ventures but loved being involved in creating memories. Sally often talked with her youthful parents about the role they would need to play in her children's lives. And she constantly reassured John that he had all the necessary attributes to be a good parent on his own. Sally also talked to all her children about her life expectancy being short and her confidence that they would thrive without her. Because Sally accepted that she was dying, no subject was left untouched.

The way she led her life highlights the vital role that the dying can play in the lives of others. Sally knew from the outset that she would die much sooner than she had expected. Accepting this, she helped others through consistent actions that celebrated a meaningful life over a long one. Her attitude permeated through the whole family and, while I wonder how many of us could carry off the feat with the same distinction, I found it a powerful thing to watch.

In her final weeks, Sally took a final holiday with her children and went to their favourite beach. Much to my frustration, she ended up in hospital there too, but nothing dented her spirits. Many people would at least mention the hiccup on their return, but she chose to talk about the fun they had.

After the holiday, her pain required more powerful drugs. When she felt weak she liked to sit in her favourite armchair by the window. She encouraged her children to stay home from school if they wished but also advised them that school could be a good distraction in such times. She had arranged to be admitted to hospice in her final days. This is where the family vigil moved, and she died peacefully, surrounded by her family, sixteen months after diagnosis.

I attended her funeral with a heavy heart. There, among other relatives, I met her ninety-year-old grandmother who lamented outliving her grand-daughter. For such a grief-filled occasion, the most extraordinary feature was the almost palpable calm in the room.

Not only had Sally talked openly about dying but she'd also been the family's anchor on the journey. And now, as every eulogy recalled, she had reminded everyone that death was universal and that they had the capacity to carry on without her. The longer I stayed the more I learnt about the great acts of kindness that Sally had quietly performed.

She had sat down with each child and spoken of her sadness while instilling them with confidence in each other and their father. She left money for her sister's unborn child, regretting they'd never meet. She bought her brother tickets to a game they had meant to watch together. She consoled her parents and asked them to care for their grandchildren. And she had even comforted her grandmother at the unfairness of losing a grandchild during her lifetime. Many people paid

Acceptance

heartfelt tributes to Sally, but her father's words stayed with me: 'She made it okay for us that she was dying.'

Witness to the most extraordinary preparation for death I had ever seen, I felt proud to have known Sally. I could almost hear her telling me that my duty to her was finished and to concentrate my energies on other patients. Leaving her funeral service, I too had the feeling that things would be okay.

I have lost more patients since Sally. Many have struggled to accept their mortality, causing consternation for them and moral distress for their carers. I am often reminded of Sally when I meet them. She found a way to live well during a terminal illness. Choosing neither unbridled optimism nor pure nihilism, she stayed on an even keel. She had a strong sense of how she wanted to live, which gave her the courage to say when she'd had enough. Her acceptance helped her avoid the desperation that prompts many people to try bizarre, unrealistic, or unsafe treatments. For someone so young, Sally packed in admirable self-knowledge and poise.

SALLY WOULD HAVE BEEN MOVED to think that her short life could provide universal lessons in dying. She would have described herself as an ordinary woman whose greatest wish was to have children and take them on lots of picnics. She wasn't a sage or a philosopher and had never had to think deeply about mortality before being forced to confront it after her holiday. But I think Sally had something many of us lack – the ability to be at one with our fate and seek to change only what lies in our control. Death was inevitable and, for her, it had come early but she could still live the best life possible. This was an exceptional attitude to bear witness to and I will always be indebted to Sally for the lessons she taught me.

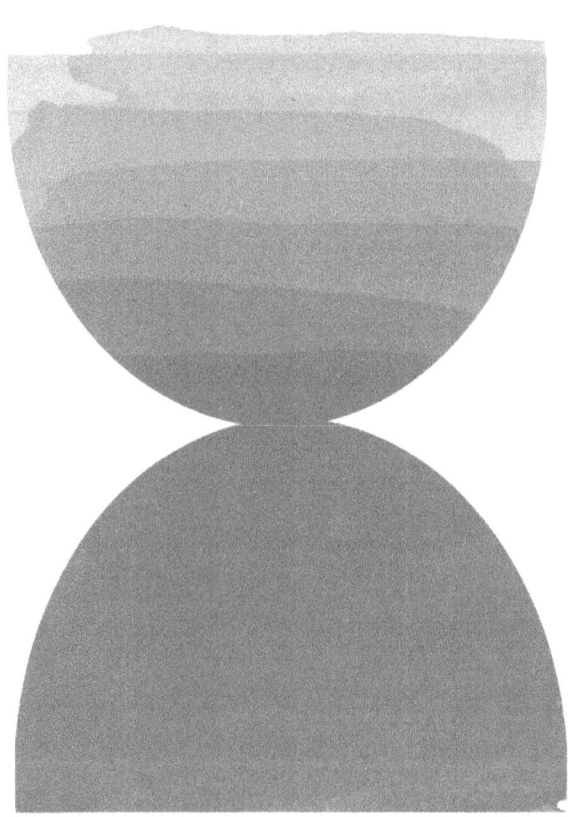

Meaning

The mystery of human existence lies not in just staying alive, but in finding something to live for.

Fyodor Dostoyevsky

THE BEST OF MEDICINE sometimes has surprisingly little to do with the medicine itself and much more with fellowship on the journey of life. The pace of modern medicine seldom permits such luxury but when it happens, it's rather special.

Charles knew he had irreversible lung disease. At just fifty, he was suffering from end-stage emphysema and was reliant on home oxygen to help him breathe. I met Charles on the ward during one of the months I worked as an internal medicine physician.

It was his sixth admission to hospital that year – a bad sign. This time, he'd contracted influenza during a particularly harsh winter.

Charles lived alone in an apartment in a nice part of town with great amenities. A successful businessman, he'd spent several years living abroad, having moved away after a relationship breakdown. He'd been stealing cigarettes from his dad since he was a boy but a wholesale renewal after the end of the relationship meant quitting smoking, curbing alcohol and taking up regular exercise. Therefore, he could hardly believe it when a series of lung infections led to the diagnosis of severe emphysema. The lung specialist thought it unusual to develop the disease at a relatively young age. He sent him to a transplant physician who warned that a lung transplant was highly complex surgery and that most patients died during the waiting period for a deceased donor to become available. By the time I met Charles, it was evident to me that he had missed his chance, but I found him clinging to the hope of receiving a new lung.

The first week in hospital was occupied by treating his influenza. The infection settled but his lungs had taken a blow and Charles was too breathless to even get out of bed. He kept hoping that he would improve in time to attend his next transplant appointment and brought this up at my daily rounds.

Charles was articulate, polite and an easy conversationalist. His smiling eyes made it even harder to deliver bad news. 'Let my transplant doctor know I'm here,' he once suggested. 'He might have some clever ideas.'

Dr Ranjana Srivastava

'We've spoken,' I assured him. 'He has no other advice than to wait for improvement.'

His disappointment was obvious.

A week later, Charles had grown even more deconditioned as a result of staying in bed. He needed a nurse to help him stand and was too breathless to participate in even gentle rehabilitation. One day, as I watched him step gingerly into the bathroom, leaning on his nurse, the truth dawned on me that Charles might not have more than a few months left to live.

'Your patient won't get home': a rehabilitation physician confirmed my fear. Up to this point, everyone had been expecting slow but eventual improvement.

Patients like Charles can easily languish in hospital if no one nudges the biggest conversations forward. I, and others, knew that we needed to broach the subject of his mortality, but his mind was a long way away, fixated on a transplant.

I wondered whether his family could help but found that he had few friends and one sister who seldom visited. From his demeanour, I very much doubted that he'd ever considered his condition to be a terminal illness. In fact, despite being bedbound for weeks, I didn't think he even understood its severity.

One day, I sat down with him as he lay propped in bed.

'Charles, I know you're waiting for things to turn around, but I'm afraid your lungs are very weak.'

'I know. I just wish they would hurry up and transplant me.'

'I think that chance has passed.'

His eyes widened.

'You really think so, doc?'

'I do.'

But before I could go on, he became distracted, making me suspect that the lack of oxygen to his brain was affecting his cognition.

The next day, I sat down with him again. This time he was attached to oxygen tubing, arranging small pieces of plastic on his bedside table.

'What's that?' I asked curiously.

'My hobby's building miniature cities and landscapes. My sister brought these in.'

I bent down to admire his neat and detailed work. It was the first time I'd seen him engaged in a task.

He was clearly delighted by my interest and I felt unkind changing the subject. He told me he still felt weak.

'Charles, I don't know if you'll get much better. We need to plan ahead.'

Instead of his usual breezy reply that he would soon get back on his feet, for the first time he gave me a pensive look.

'Do you think I'm dying?' he finally asked, taking me by surprise.

'I think you are,' I said, filled with regret but also relieved that we had reached this stage.

'But I'm not done with life,' he protested. 'I have so many ideas in my head.'

His lament spoke to me because my own head is constantly churning with ideas that I always assume I will have time for later.

He continued wryly, 'I thought you had to be eighty or ninety to think about meaning. I'm only fifty.'

I didn't know what to say. So, I simply listened to him as he formed his own correct view that he was dying, and I saw how just allowing his thoughts to unfold brought about a thus-far-elusive realisation. Charles acknowledged the short time he had left and declared that absent further useful interventions, he'd like to leave hospital and enjoy building his miniature cities. He had us cancel his various respiratory appointments.

The social worker found him a nursing home close to his sister. It was a sad day seeing Charles leave, as he was one of the nicest patients I'd ever met. He gladly greeted my team each morning like long-lost friends. Although we constantly delivered bad news, he never withheld a compliment and frequently told us how fortunate patients were to be under our care. His words were like balm to his providers, who often fought their own emotions at the unfairness of his situation.

Every eye in the room was moist as he shook hands with the team and told us he'd miss us.

Charles contracted another infection and died in his sleep three months later. His sister marvelled that he was a changed man in that time. He stopped hoping for a turnaround, embraced his relationships, enjoyed good food and wine, and wrote a generous will, forgetting no one. He gave away his prized miniature collections to a little boy who used to visit his grandmother in the nursing home and always peeked in to see what Charles was building next. He left a fine reading lamp to a nurse who was a former refugee and who practised speaking English with him. He never failed to tell his sister how much he loved their long car trips when they reminisced over their lives. According to everyone who met him, there were countless such gestures of goodwill as his health deteriorated. Charles had always had a streak of kindness in him but reconciling with mortality had magnified it.

His sister warmly reflected that her successful and ambitious brother had fretted over finding the meaning of life, reminding me of his lament in hospital, but she thought he had found it in a hundred small acts of consideration. This reminded me of Ralph Waldo Emerson's words: 'The purpose of life is to be useful, to be honourable, to be compassionate, to have it make some difference that you have lived and lived well.'

Our exchange prompted me to wonder how any of us finds meaning in life. Would I myself scramble to create it or would there be a pre-existing stock waiting to be unwrapped? How and when do we find meaning in life? What does meaning feel like? Who gets to think of meaning?

Meaning can seem like a towering concept better suited to the intellectuals among us, or perhaps those who have time to gaze at the ocean and contemplate the minutiae of life, than ordinary people. Most days, it is more than enough to manage our daily needs of buying groceries, paying bills, finding childcare and employment. It might even strike some as mildly indulgent to contemplate what imbues our lives with deeper meaning – and I suspect that most of us wouldn't even know where to begin. But in fact, the search for meaning is hardly an intellectual exercise, it's a thoroughly practical one. To identify our values, our motivations, and what lies at our core is essential to dying well.

I have learnt this from years of working in a metropolitan hospital with a high share of socially disadvantaged and impoverished people, asylum seekers and refugees. My patients are not academics, intellectuals or philosophers; many have no formal education. Some have indescribably difficult stressors running through their entire life before they become seriously ill. But when it comes to finding purpose and meaning, there seems to be little correlation with status, income, or age. Those who acquit themselves well have often accepted the vagaries of fate and focus on their own actions. It's instructive to see how they remain calm amid trying circumstances and a lot has to do with knowing what matters.

I once cared for a patient, Maya, whose sensible exchanges put every doctor at ease. She was on the ward after sustaining a severe heart attack and when asked about her views on resuscitation, replied, 'I have lived through a lot. If you feel you can help me, I'd like you to do what you can. If you think I am dying, I'm ready to go.' The distinction she drew between staying well and merely existing without quality of life was clear and wise and yet Maya had never finished school. After fleeing war, she'd spent her life working on a factory line where she met her husband, yet she could encapsulate the meaning of her life in one word – family. She told me she was proud to have raised four children with seven professional degrees between them. In a life that could have taunted her with abundant missed opportunities, Maya chose simplicity. She regretted that she had never had the chance to study and prove herself but derived frank happiness from the achievements of her children and grandchildren. 'I want to live forever to enjoy them, but I will die knowing my job is done.' To hear Maya satisfied was to be satisfied.

She survived without needing resuscitation, but her heart function did not restore itself. She went downhill over a period of months, able to exert herself less and less. So, when I received a call from a community nurse, I could confidently say that Maya was ready to die with the least possible fuss. The nurse started a morphine infusion and Maya died peacefully. Though her passing was sad, it was consoling for everyone to know she had lived and died happily, as she had herself said many times.

Another memorable patient, Hugh, undertook a unique search for meaning. Hugh came from a distinguished family and when I met him in hospice, he told me that his grandfather and father, both eminent judges, had written widely on important judicial matters. In his late forties and himself a judge, Hugh had embarked on a memoir about the two legendary figures in his life when he'd fallen ill unexpectedly. He knew that time was running out and he wanted to finish his book as a tribute to his family and a gift to his children. As a writer, I was intrigued, never previously having met a dying man racing to the finish of his book. I learnt a remarkable lesson in perseverance and promise. Hugh woke up early and used his saved strength to type his manuscript. On days he didn't feel like typing, he dictated, and his large family took turns at the keyboard. I wondered sometimes whether his wife and children resented his preoccupation, but I saw that finishing the book became the family's joint mission. It fuelled them and brought them together. It was both their way of grieving and of celebrating and his room frequently rang with laughter while overflowing with dictionaries and references. For this family, it was too hard to make sense of fate, but they found meaning through writing.

Hugh managed to write a complete draft and the family had it beautifully bound. It rested at his bedside and he told me that whenever he felt sad about dying, he thought of the book as his legacy. Hugh's loss was forever accompanied by a sense of victory at his and his family's extraordinary achievement.

The common thread in dying well is the capacity to find meaning in things big and small. These days, it's common to receive treatment towards the end of life but I see that most discerning patients never invest all hope in the outcome and are deliberately mindful about quality of life, even when it means upsetting those who don't agree. Instead of dwelling on what could go wrong, they take continuous stock of their lives. Their blessings might range from a long marriage to healthy children, a few close friends, a thriving beehive, a flourishing garden or a late-life companion. Where gratitude abounds, meaning thrives.

It's not that their lives have no missteps or tragedy but even from these, they have learnt something about themselves or the world. One of my favourite patients recently asked me to stop her treatment. Since her divorce, she and her children had been especially close, and she was determined to attend her son's wedding. The break allowed her to conserve enough energy to attend the ceremony with a front-row seat and enjoy much pampering. Less than twenty-four hours later, she was brought to hospital in an unconscious state. The emergency doctors couldn't believe she had survived the wedding, but I wasn't surprised. She had known what mattered and gone to great lengths to make it happen. Consequently, she gave her son the best wedding gift of all: her presence.

I have seen through the eyes of many patients that the things that give meaning to our lives need not be public, popular or impressive. Indeed, they should be enough to console us and our loved ones that our lives have been worthwhile. Being insistently familiar with our purpose in life doesn't banish all regret but it cushions our falls. This is why it's never too early to start thinking about what a meaningful life looks like for ourselves.

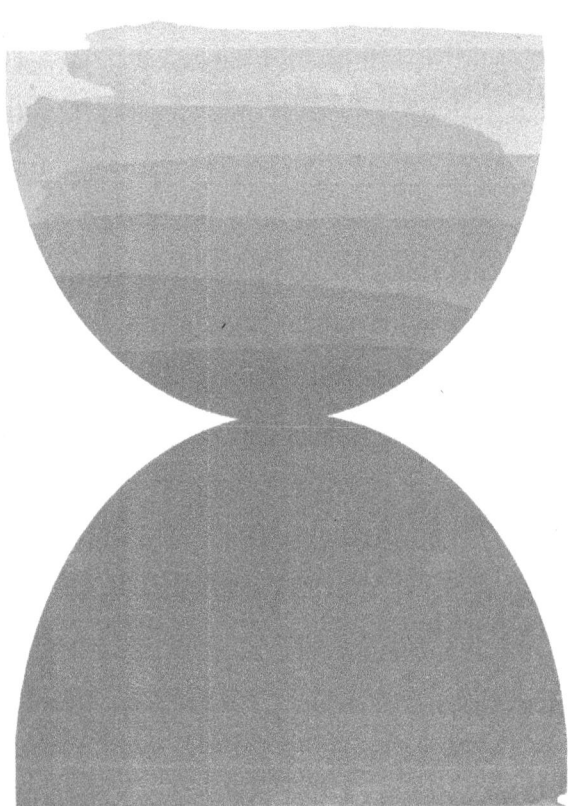

Forgiveness

*Home is where you are loved the most
and act the worst.*

Marjorie Pay Hinckley

'SHE'S GROWING THIN and her stomach pains won't go away, so the doctor has sent her for some sort of a scan,' reported my friend Leela, an artist who had mostly lived her life among talented, healthy people. Unused to the realm of medicine, she didn't realise how much her words chilled me. We had gone to school together and I'd grown up watching her mother consuming cigarettes as if they were food.

Leela's mother had an affair that led to the breakdown of an anaemic marriage. Her father moved out and found love in the arms of a very distant cousin, which proved socially excruciating. The subsequent relationship between her parents was acrimonious and volatile, and rather than dissipating with time, it got worse. To protect herself, Leela quietly distanced herself from both parents and went abroad for a few years, only to return home to a battle that had never ceased. She was aghast at the contempt she was surrounded by and often rued her dysfunctional family. Nonetheless, she strived to maintain a relationship with both parents, something that she increasingly valued after she became a parent to twins. Sadly, the relationship never achieved the harmony she was after. Leela's closest contact was her brother but he lived in another city with his family.

Against this backdrop of stress, Leela's mother was confirmed as having advanced cancer and I waited with dismay to see what would happen next. The news affected everyone differently. Her mother was sanguine, Leela and her brother were shocked, and their father showed no outward emotion.

Leela accompanied her mother to the oncologist, who was truthful and sensitive. He told them he would do everything possible but the chance of a sustained response to treatment was small. Leela's mother enquired about her prognosis and when he replied between six to nine months, she was floored. Seized by a fervour to beat the odds, she began chemotherapy but most noticeable was a change in her outlook: she began taking stock of her life.

Assuming this amounted to clearing her debts and writing a will, Leela was surprised when her mother repeatedly expressed a wish to see the family together. She waited for her mother to change her tune but when she didn't, Leela arranged lunch at her house.

Leela's parents were meeting again after many years and it would also be the first time her mother met her ex-husband's new partner. I winced at the disaster that could be in the making. As if reading my thoughts, Leela called me.

'It was quite nice,' she reported. 'Everyone behaved well and there was genuine concern and sympathy for Mum.'

The family was so complicated that I found this fascinating. I asked about her father and she told me he'd been mostly quiet because he felt bad. He'd offered to take her mother to her appointments and she had said she'd consider it. Leela added that her mother had kept up a brave face in front of the others but when they'd left, she had clung to her and broken into sobs. Her mother had always been spirited and combative and to see another side of her was confronting. Later, Leela's father had called her to confess his guilt that the divorce had exacerbated his ex-wife's smoking habit. Meanwhile, Leela's younger brother was still processing things, worried that there wasn't the time for any fruitful reconciliation.

I sympathised with the emotional storm engulfing Leela, who after all had no preparation for handling such a complex situation. Sadly, her mother only lived six months past her diagnosis, but in those months, I was privileged to watch the profound healing that people are capable of.

The family dynamics were undeniably messy. The stress of a terminal illness can unleash people's worse tendencies, but this was a family determined to make the last few months count.

Leela's father voluntarily apologised for the hurt he had caused his ex-wife. Listening to, and acknowledging, his ex-wife's remorse was also helpful. His second wife was polite but stayed out of major family discussions. Prudently, she offered neither effusive friendship nor solicitous concern but encouraged her husband to do what he needed.

Leela requested flexible working hours and attended every appointment with her mother. Her brother had a much harder time warming to their mother but supported Leela. He became her confidant as they discussed the changes in their mother, who had gone from being disillusioned and dismissive to shedding much of her judgmental side. Their conversations unearthed strong feelings and regret that they often struggled to understand. More than once Leela sighed that it would have been easier to lose their 'other' mother.

I saw Leela's mother once or twice and reassured her that she was in capable hands. She told me that she was apprehensive of the future but felt secure around her family, confessing that she felt undeserving of their support. However, it was gratifying to see how their support sustained her.

I also know from my conversations with Leela what intense emotion swirled beneath the family's newfound equilibrium. She felt cheated that just as she had gained the maturity to put the past behind her, her time with her mother had been slashed. Her brother was hurting that his future children wouldn't get to know their grandmother and they both relived their disappointment at being let down by their parents. Compassion didn't come naturally under those circumstances but the catharsis it brought was evident. It was impressive to watch the family put forgiveness first, because the topic comes up all too often for my patients at the end of life. Pride is an important part of our makeup but when we let pride rule us, we can't make appropriate decisions for ourselves and those we hold dear. Misplaced pride prevents us from making amends, understanding different perspectives and meeting others in the middle. Forgiveness turns out to be a noble concept that's difficult to implement but it's a cause worth pursuing for its rich rewards.

It is rightly said that trust takes years to build, a moment to destroy and a lifetime to rebuild. Leela's mother wisely understood that she could not take back her mistakes but what she got right was to graciously accept even the smallest gestures her family made. Whereas she would previously have thumbed her nose at a regular lunch or a nightly phone call, now she welcomed it. Her genuine remorse fuelled her motivation to change what she could in her limited time. The hardest and most significant thing she did was to sit down with both her children to explain aspects of her conduct that had hurt them and ask for their forgiveness. Leela described this as the most powerful amend she made and the most consoling memory.

Before Leela's mother died, the siblings spent weeks caring for her at home, something they did not foresee at her diagnosis. Although those weeks could not replace lost time, they were therapeutic and memorable. Her relationship with her ex-husband was cordial without being cloying. She acknowledged his pain, described hers and openly forgave him. To hear her say this was a turning point in his life opened the way for them to discuss their hopes for their children and grandchildren, a meaningful rite of passage.

The last time I saw Leela's mother, she looked tired, but I thought that her tumultuous life had moved to a calmer place. She had fulfilled some personal wishes and reconciled with the most important people in her life, her family. Her contentment was mixed with humility, as if she accepted responsibility for some actions.

I was inspired to see that a difficult road had led to a hopeful future. At her funeral, there was sadness but also recognition that our lives can be enriched by forgiveness and reconciliation.

It has been eye-opening for me to see that the way we treat each other is critical to dying well. Death is insufficient to erase our reservations about a fraught marriage, a tense friendship or a broken bond; unresolved tensions cause enduring harm. Leela's family shows us that the power to forgive ourselves, forgive others and repair relationships lies within us all. When confronted by troubled relationships at the end of life, we might try to remember that the wounds of love are best healed by those who made them.

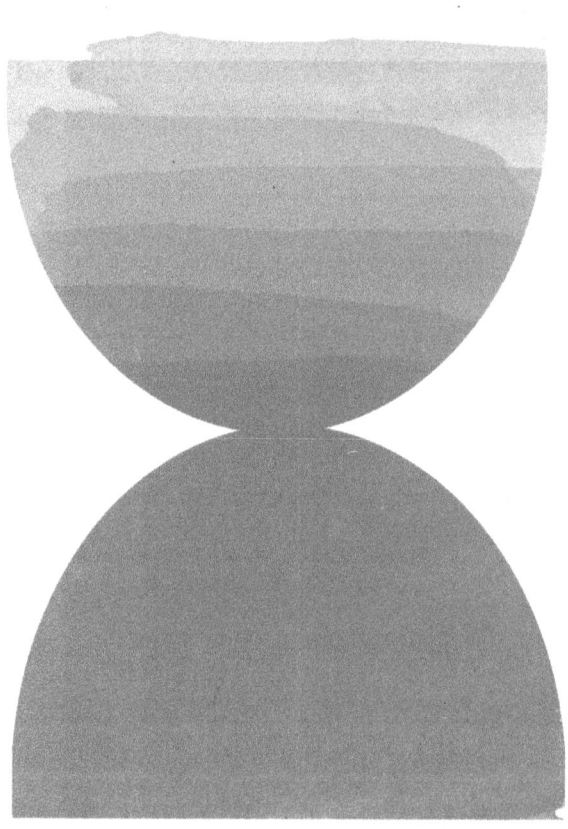

Equanimity

Equanimity is calamity's medicine.
Publilius Syrus

Of all the qualities I observe in my patients, I'm most attracted to equanimity; that calmness and composure some people demonstrate, especially in difficult situations. Equanimity interests me because I routinely see how people who acquit themselves with calm fare better in almost every walk of life and, unsurprisingly, in death. The capacity to retreat into an inner sanctum of calm is one of the greatest gifts we can hope to possess amid the hype of medicine and the noise of life.

Occasional unruly emotions and disorganised thoughts are common at the end of life, but if they become persistent, they can be very troubling for the patient and taxing for caregivers.

A common worry of many terminally ill patients focuses on a specific subject: how to avoid dying. In turn, this translates into a very difficult question for doctors: what can medicine do to prevent death? To face the finality of death is no ordinary task even for the most prepared among us, but the task is much harder when we are primed by circumstances for most of our lives to deny the thought of death.

We are all influenced by the breathless media reports of miracles and breakthroughs that paint death as the ultimate failure. Uncertain how to handle the topic, we shield our children from it and avoid discussing it with our friends. Even in a workplace like mine, where death might be thought to feature openly, it mostly isn't. We spend our lives curiously, knowing that everyone dies but unable to draw closer to our own mortality. Partly, this is necessary, for if we were to continuously dwell on death, we would not achieve much in life. However, failing to reckon at all with our mortality risks living a life devoid of meaning. But with its seemingly unlimited offer of drugs and interventions, combined with a reluctance to view our lives as limited, modern medicine makes equanimity in death harder than ever.

If the duty of a doctor goes beyond diagnosing and prescribing and encompasses the task of helping people live and die well, by far the most challenging part of my job is addressing the existential distress of patients who cannot accept that they are dying. If their fears can be resolved, it feels like time well spent. If they are not, the disquiet is very hard to shake. Perhaps this is why it's easy to be drawn to patients who are composed, even poised, about their death. Among doctors, nurses, and even other patients, they are regarded with respect and awe because I think we all wish we could be like them.

Paul was in his fifties when he was diagnosed with lung cancer. There is such stigma attached to the diagnosis that he took pains to reassure me that he had never touched a cigarette in his life. I believed him and saw the unfairness through his eyes.

Sometimes a moment becomes frozen in our mind – it was like this at my first meeting with Paul. I remember the room and the bed he was in and how he leant towards one side because his other side hurt. He had arrived the night before with pain thought to be related to kidney stones but a short while later scan results would devastate him and his wife, Laura. Cancer dotted his spine – the excruciating pain in his side had nothing to do with stones but widespread bone metastases. But where had they come from? Paul had to endure another wait before tests confirmed him to have advanced lung cancer.

Fit, healthy and at the peak of his career, Paul was stunned by the diagnosis and thought there must be a mistake.

'I don't smoke,' he frowned.

'I know, but some non-smokers develop lung cancer too,' I sympathised, feeling as hollow as my explanation.

Laura sat at Paul's feet on the narrow bed as they listened carefully to the new language of cancer. His tumour profile meant that he could be spared chemotherapy in favor of a pill, which had fewer side effects.

'I'll follow your instructions to the letter,' Paul promised.

'We're putting our faith in you, doctor,' Laura pleaded.

Their world had been upturned in twenty-four hours, but they were calm on the exterior.

From that day on, Paul kept his word despite all the ups and downs. He responded very well to treatment; the cancer shrank and his pains eased, lifting all our spirits. I fervently hoped that the medication would see him through to a time when even better drugs became available. With cancer medicine moving at breakneck speed, new and effective treatments are announced regularly.

For nearly eight months, Paul stayed largely well and worked full-time. Occasionally, he had pain, nausea and insomnia as well as an angry rash but in all the time I knew him he never once complained about his fate. He intuitively appreciated that he was better off than many others and drew a certain consolation from this.

Paul was an experienced migration professional who took pride in helping people navigate the complexities of the migration process. A migrant himself, he understood the stress and emotion involved and took great care to accompany people on the journey. He once told me that although our jobs differed, people also came to him with hope and it was his duty to treat them with compassion. I was moved by the comparison and not at all surprised to hear about Paul's popularity at work.

The hardest thing about looking after people who are adored by family and colleagues alike is getting to know them well while knowing that their reprieve will have an end. When Paul's pain re-surfaced and he complained of feeling weak, my fears of disease progression were confirmed. Paul took the news with his customary equanimity and asked what was next.

By a stroke of luck, a brand-new pill became available, whose efficacy looked extremely promising. I grasped at the thought of extending Paul's life by another year or more, which might sound bleak unless one realised that the average life expectancy in advanced lung cancer is measured in months.

My enthusiasm doubled when another oncologist marvelled how the drug had melted away his patient's disease. With a bow to modern medicine, I told Paul about the drug.

Since I had always been honest with him, I made it clear that it wouldn't cure him but hopefully would keep his disease at bay for many months.

'I trust you,' he simply said. 'I know you'll do your best.'

His words would follow me for the rest of his life.

Equanimity

I would have doubted it had I not seen it myself, but almost overnight his pain vanished and he felt better. The emotional release of such unexpected results is indescribable.

I will never forget the memory of an ecstatic Paul and a relieved Laura sharing my hope that the drug would work as long as it took for something even better to arrive. I encouraged them to make plans that they had kept putting on hold.

And then, as suddenly as it had started to work, within weeks the tide turned. Paul came to hospital feeling weak and tired and his condition kept deteriorating. Doctors, including me, racked their brains until it became obvious that the drug had stopped working and Paul was dying. Paul and I talked daily during this time. He asked questions to refine his understanding, but never expressed frustration, anger or doubt about what was happening to him. My own mind was in knots those days, desperately wondering where I went wrong – Paul's composure was as reassuring as it was inspiring.

There were many tears shed on the day Paul went into hospice. He went there willingly and died in the presence of his large extended family and his loyal dog.

Hearing the news of his hourly decline, I had rushed to visit him and was dismayed to see him so changed. He had trouble moving in bed, but his eyes lit up at seeing me and he greeted me with the same warmth and generosity of spirit as he had all year long. He introduced me to the rest of his family and thanked me for my care, which seemed ironic because I felt that care had failed him too early. The day before he died, I was astonished to find him lucid and completely prepared to die.

'It's in God's hands now,' he said softly as I held his thin hand. 'I've had a very good life and you did your best.'

Many people would have expressed regret but here was Paul absolving me of any guilt.

Most astonishing, however, was the sheer calm that filled the room as a result of Paul's equanimity. People came and went quietly, unafraid to look at him and say a quiet word. There were tears but also ordinary conversations. His dog lay quietly on the floor, as if sensing the solemnity of the occasion. A nurse came to check if he was comfortable. At Paul's praise of her care, she broke into a smile. As she insightfully observed, it was rare to see patients play such an outsized role in their own peaceful death.

When Paul died, I felt his loss acutely and attended his packed funeral to pay my respects. The church was filled with mourners – he didn't lack those who loved him. I sat in the back and listened to people's memories of him. From the pastor to his friends, everyone hailed Paul's generosity of spirit. They mentioned his capacity for love and his ability to forgive, but most of all they talked about the same quality that had stayed with me: his enduring calm in the face of impending death. Paul hadn't denied his circumstances, he'd just been determined not to let them bring him down. Hearing people speak, I felt lucky to have known Paul and learnt something from him about accepting mortality. I saw how his genuine care for others enriched his own end-of-life experience because people instinctively gave back more than they received.

Laura told me that Paul's religion had been his anchor, which made me think of how uncommon this is in an increasingly secular world. A devout churchgoer, Paul never advertised his religion but it was evident that his equanimity stemmed in no small part from his deeply held faith. We all desire purpose and for Paul religion was part of his purpose. While we may be living in an era where even the mention of religion can create awkwardness, I saw how religion can shape our thoughts and help cultivate calm. My heart ached when Laura lamented that even the dog missed Paul's equanimity.

Paul could have been forgiven for adopting a very different attitude. His unsuspected diagnosis and unsuccessful treatment could have been a breeding ground for resentment. Patients in Paul's situation can be the most bitter – never able to overcome the betrayal of their body, their hopes and their future. Sometimes, by expressing our natural sympathy, we can unintentionally aggravate their bitterness. Paul attracted many well-wishers who suggested ways to cure his cancer and it's surprising he tolerated them all, but his innate calm told him that they meant well.

Dr Ranjana Srivastava

I had a chance to interview Laura and their two daughters for a radio program I made about the ripple effect of cancer and was curious to learn how Paul spent the last few months of his life. I heard that he located as many friends and family members as he could to request their forgiveness for past wrongs. Apparently, no one could think of such an instance, which shows the measure of the man.

Having promised to buy his daughter her first car, he took the time to find something safe and appealing. He spent hours with Laura, patiently coaching her on how to deal with the paperwork his death would generate, even building her a spreadsheet with the details. 'He would simply say, "If anything were to happen, this is what I want you to do."'

In the family's telling, Paul filled his life with so many meaningful things that there was no room for anger or regret. As we spoke, I sensed their equanimity and couldn't help reflecting on the impact of one person on an entire family's outlook.

Paul's death left a vacuum in my office. Doctors must move on to tend their other patients but Paul's conduct gave me great food for thought.

One of the most quoted works of Indian mythology, the *Bhagavad Gita*, is based on the exchange on the battlefield between Arjuna, a gifted warrior, and his mentor, Lord Krishna. As he surveys the ready armies on both sides, Arjuna is overcome by grief and concern for the losses he is about to incur and inflict. Krishna encourages him with the following advice: 'Wherever the mind wanders, restless and diffuse in its search for satisfaction without, lead it within; train it to rest in the Self.'

We have been encouraged since ancient times to make an effort to seek calm. Paul's remarkable capacity to train the mind to rest in the self contains wisdom for us all.

Dr Ranjana Srivastava

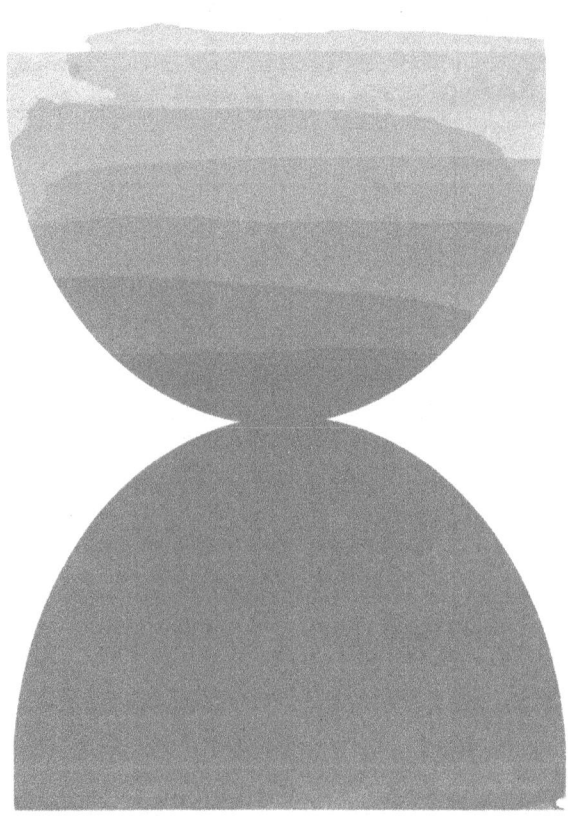

Kindness

*A part of kindness consists in loving people
more than they deserve.*

Joseph Joubert

ONE OF THE HARDEST QUESTIONS doctors confront is not what treatment to prescribe, but what to do about the simple things that can quickly derail people's welfare, especially at the end of life. Even in the wealthiest societies, these issues often have to do with food, shelter, money and support. Hospitals can help for a time, but it is often beyond their capacity to address the root cause.

Looking after patients affected by poverty, violence or neglect and then caught in the tangle of bureaucracy is challenging. But it doesn't have to be so complicated — I meet plenty of patients who lead a completely stable life until a serious illness reveals the faultlines and they are left feeling vulnerable and alone.

When these problems occur at the end of life, the urgency to solve them is even greater. In such instances, kindness can arise from the most unexpected quarters, lightening the load for patients and doctors and creating good memories for others.

Sarah was a twenty-six-year-old student and part-time nanny I met in hospital after her year-long struggle against a rare neurological condition that even experts had difficulty pinpointing. Over a two-month stay in hospital, I watched her cognitive and physical capacity deteriorate. She was steadily losing weight, was often drowsy and sometimes confused, and needed increasing help to manage core activities such as feeding and showering. It became clear that her poor prognosis was inalterable.

On a ward round Sarah told me that she'd had an inkling from the outset that she had a life-limiting disease and expressed her wish to go home and live out the remainder of her life in familiar surroundings. She missed her dog and the small garden she had planted in a box in her tiny apartment. Uncomfortable at how long Sarah had spent in hospital with no meaningful gain, I was delighted at the prospect of sending her home with support from the community palliative care team. Except our plans hit an early roadblock. Sarah could no longer afford to pay rent and even if she could, her upstairs apartment was unsuitable for access. Sarah was an immigrant whose family still lived abroad. She thought about going back home but her palliative care needs were determined to be too complex to be met in her home country which, like most of the world, lacked access to morphine, oxygen and other palliative care essentials. In order to be discharged, Sarah needed a home and a carer – even the best-equipped hospital would be hard-pressed to furnish these.

Amid these serious challenges, the first thing that impressed me was Sarah's kindness towards her providers. She accepted her illness but was greatly concerned for the staff working long shifts, especially when she found out they had skipped a meal. On these occasions, she'd encourage them to look after themselves and offer to wait to be seen. Although the staff always put her needs first, the gesture touched them greatly. I couldn't help noticing that Sarah was even kind to the other patients, who were all older and in better health than her. Before it became too hard, she would read the newspaper aloud to the elderly patient in the next bed. Sarah's kindness softened us all. When people see our best qualities, we strive to deserve it.

I knew that as long as she stayed in hospital she wouldn't lack genuine affection; nonetheless, she needed to go home.

The social worker was looking everywhere for assistance and a staff member had just begun enquiring if she could house Sarah when Sarah's former employer, Ina, called us. Ina was a young academic who had relied on Sarah to look after her son while she completed her thesis. She had heard about Sarah's illness through a mutual friend and guiltily enquired whether she had missed any signs. I reassured her that Sarah's decline had been quite sudden and when she expressed concern about her prolonged hospitalisation, I mentioned the dilemma.

'Sarah doesn't have a home to go to,' I explained. 'The social worker is exploring possibilities, but everything takes time. Your visits may help Sarah.'

'I want to do more,' Ina replied.

Just hours later she called the social worker to say that she and her husband were prepared to care for Sarah. The social worker was sceptical about a young couple with a child coping with the care of a terminally ill patient not much older than them. But Ina explained that they had been greatly aided by Sarah in their time of need and felt that caring for her was the right thing to do.

'She'd have done the same for us,' Ina remarked.

I was moved by her gesture and happy for Sarah but cautiously advised that we would need to look at the logistics and Sarah would obviously have to agree.

Social work and palliative care thought the solution was tenable and Sarah, facing the prospect of indefinite hospitalisation, was overjoyed. A few days later, Sarah left hospital and the nurse who visited her at home told me that she had rarely met a more confident couple willing to undertake the onerous task of caring for someone at the end of life.

Although I would never see Sarah again, I kept track of her progress. True to their word, Ina and her husband ensured she had everything she needed, including the company of her dog. They also accepted help from another academic couple. Since Sarah spent most of her time in bed, the academics worked from home while providing her with quiet company.

I heard that Ina and her husband had done a great job of explaining things to their young son who was confidently involved in small but important tasks such as filling Sarah's water jug and making her bed.

One day, Ina called me to say that although Sarah never mentioned it, it was clear that she longed to see her parents.

'They speak every day, but do you think there's time to fly them here?'

Surprised, I advised that time was running out but also that the logistics would be arduous. Nonetheless, I wrote a letter to the immigration department and Ina's friends organised a fundraiser which provided enough money to fly her parents to her bedside.

Everyone involved was gratified at the compassion shown to Sarah, which disproved the common belief that the world is too self-absorbed to care about others. But my education hardly ended there.

Ina's house was just large enough to accommodate Sarah but left no room for her parents. At this point, Ina's elderly neighbour appeared with an offer to house Sarah and her parents in her spacious, mostly unoccupied home. She had heard about Sarah's predicament and wanted to help.

It would have been impossible to script a better story and the neighbour's gesture gave fresh meaning to 'the kindness of strangers'.

The volunteers continued to look after Sarah as she became less mobile and comforted her parents by listening to them reminisce. They learnt how to administer her medication and when to call for help. The nurses were full of praise for how the volunteers thrived on being useful, but never overwhelmed Sarah or her parents with their kindness. 'It's like they were born to do this,' one marvelled.

I wasn't surprised to learn that Sarah was openly grateful to all her carers. Her restlessness in hospital had been replaced by ease. While she avoided the topic of dying, she accepted her decline and exuded a quiet confidence that she was in safe hands. A nurse reflected that for a woman so young, Sarah was a thoughtful patient who knew the importance of acknowledging her helpers. She recognised if they looked tired, asked after their children and made sure they knew how much she appreciated their sacrifices. For the carers, it was enough to be thanked.

In her last days, Sarah went to a hospice, where she died peacefully. Her young volunteers were sobered by her death but took rightful pride in their ability to join together and help in a way they had never imagined. They humbly reflected that it had been a life-changing experience for them which had made them appreciate their own good fortune.

I often think about Sarah and Ina and the way they illuminated the lives of others with their remarkable kindness. Their conduct was a lesson in practising kindness even when we may feel limited by our circumstances.

We can be challenged by the act of dying and the act of caring for the dying. In both cases, behaving with kindness towards others can be an antidote to our preoccupations – in fact, there are few things more transformative. I'm routinely humbled by the capacity of my patients to be kind to me while contending with their own weighty issues. They ask after my children, write a kind note, or bring honey from their collection. Their kindness spurs me on to be a better doctor and a better person. Well-wishers often ask me how best to help the dying. The answer is often quite simple: by being present and by being kind. My patients often wish someone would read aloud to them, help them write letters and record a legacy. Almost everyone I meet would be overjoyed to have someone just sit quietly with them, which may be the greatest act of easing the loneliness of dying. Kindness need not be loud and overwhelming, only consoling.

All too often we underestimate the power of small gestures but in debating how best to be kind, we would do well to be persuaded by Oscar Wilde's remark that the smallest act of kindness is worth more than the grandest intention.

Dr Ranjana Srivastava

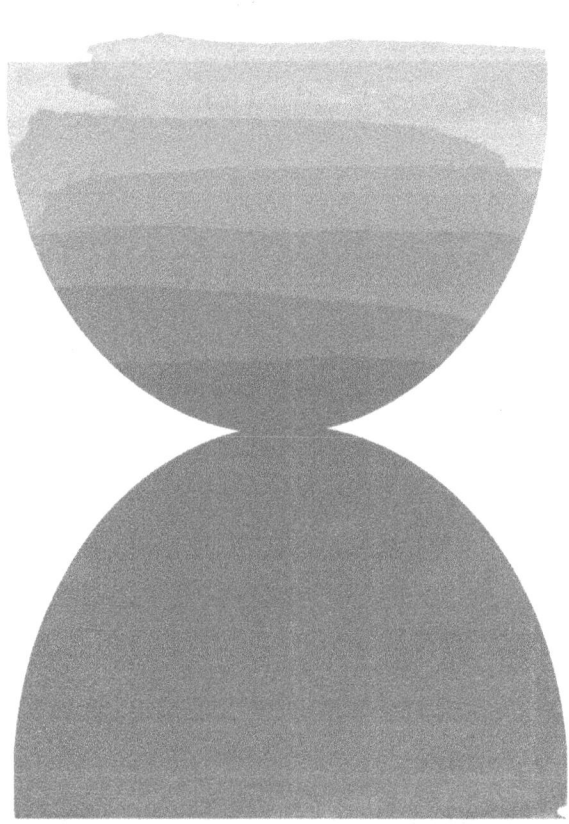

Gratitude

If the only prayer you ever say in your entire life is thank you, it will be enough.

Meister Eckhart

I AM PASSIONATE ABOUT BEING A DOCTOR, but some days I feel as if the world, to quote the poet Yeats, is 'more full of weeping than you can understand'. Many of my patients are old, sick and helpless, with children who are themselves sick, busy or simply unavailable. Even younger patients with a terminal illness have often been cast adrift from the personal and societal connections they might otherwise have. One can't help but be struck by the physical, emotional and existential concerns faced by the dying, but the story of medicine would be incomplete without mentioning all the people who find the capacity to conduct themselves with grace, composure and, most of all, gratitude. In my view, this is one of the best parts of being a doctor.

Although one might think it unusual in an era of instant gratification, there are people who never bemoan their fate. They don't downplay their problems, they ask probing questions and challenge doctors' verdicts but they defy the notion that all dying must be dramatic or complicated. At a time in life so commonly associated with a lack of control, there is no doubt that they are in charge. They strike me as resilient and pragmatic, but if I had to pick their most important invisible underlying trait, it would be gratitude.

These are people who, over the course of their life, have catalogued all kinds of reasons to be grateful. When nearing the end of life, their most consequential choices are illuminated by the same approach. My most grateful patients have made things easier for themselves and their caregivers. And I can't mention gratitude without recalling Ian, another one of my favorite patients.

It was a busy day and Ian had been kept waiting. Many of my patients recall their first appointment with absolute clarity and I often wish that the most significant appointments in a patient's life, such as when they discover a diagnosis or receive serious test results, could run like clockwork, but unfortunately, this rarely happens because human beings have feelings.

The patient before Ian had suddenly crumpled under the weight of her circumstances and there was no way to wrap up the consultation on time. By the time I had calmed her, found a nurse, and called her husband, I was running considerably late. I remember accompanying Ian and his family from the waiting room and apologising for the delay.

'The last patient needed a bit more time,' I explained.

'It's okay, I imagine everyone here needs more time,' Ian responded lightly and I was instantly moved by his consideration.

At seventy-one, he had recently retired from his job as a baker, joking that after forty years in the business it was time to see why people liked sleeping in. The small community had bid him a fond farewell as he handed over the reins to his grandson. Ian took his first extended holiday with his wife and came back feeling unwell. He teased her that unemployment didn't agree with him but she insisted on tests.

In the room, I explained to Ian that the surgeon had skilfully removed his cancer and now he required a course of chemotherapy to reduce the risk of recurrence. Sobered by his diagnosis, he told me he wanted to do everything possible to stay healthy in the next phase of his life.

Ian quickly became known for his friendly demeanour. Early on, his nurse commented that a life of customer service had really given him the ability to read people. He could interpret body language and was pleasant without being intrusive. I thought her description apt.

In clinic, he was polite and unassuming. He brushed off the frequent blood tests and long waits as minor inconveniences and never failed to say thank you. What I especially liked about Ian was his clear sense of what was important to him. He told me very early that he valued his independence and quality of life and would rather stop treatment than live to regret the toxicities.

Although conscious of the sheer number of appointments he had to keep, I looked forward to Ian's visits. He always came with his wife, and at least one of his five children. Having watched so many patients navigate this difficult time in their lives alone or with unreliable support, I grew to admire his close-knit family. But I could also see that, despite his openness, a part of his life belonged only to him. He was interested in people's opinions but everyone knew who made the final decision. At a time when so many people feel jostled by their circumstances, his composure seemed all the more admirable.

I was dumbstruck when Ian's cancer returned within months of finishing treatment.

Again, I walked Ian and his wife down the corridor to my office, their tension palpable.

I got straight to the point, as he would want. My heart ached as I explained the implications of the recurrence and discussed treatment options that might extend his life but not cure him. Ian's usual ebullient expression turned pensive.

'All that treatment did no good,' he said quietly.

'It looks like that,' I sighed. 'I'm sorry.'

It's tempting for a doctor to fill the quiet space left in the wake of grim pronouncements with new promises, but I waited to take Ian's cue, wondering whether his calm would finally collapse. I should have given him more credit.

When he finally spoke, he said, 'I can't imagine how hard it must be for you to give this news.'

I was speechless that a man reeling from bad news would find room in his heart for someone else. Ian's wife regarded him with the same admiration that I felt.

The nurses were dismayed to hear Ian's news. They found that, although he was still friendly, he had grown more serious. During his previous visits, there was the end of treatment to look forward to, but now that was gone, his future hanging in the balance.

He started chemotherapy and we settled into a new routine. He didn't like to dwell on his terminal illness, instead choosing to talk about other things.

The first diagnosis of cancer had sobered him, but its recurrence prompted him to prioritise. He was a keen craftsman who had kept up his woodwork hobby even in the busiest periods of his life. Now he'd decided to rejuvenate his workshop for some large projects, starting with a dining table for his youngest daughter, the only one of his children he hadn't done this for.

'How long will that take?' I asked out of curiosity, instantly regretting he would think me out of place for questioning his prognosis.

'In my current state, a couple of months, but I'm happy to be doing it,' he said, smiling.

I cheered him on until I saw the pictures of the finished product completed in record time. Next, he made his wife a fruit bowl. Admiring its polish and exquisite workmanship, I couldn't help asking how he felt while making these pieces. He answered as if he'd frequently thought about it.

'Sometimes I'm sad that my workshop will end with me. But mostly, I focus on the joy it brings people. I like making things that will stay with my family.'

I thought then of how the consolations of a legacy came so readily to some.

He mentioned his wife's fear that he would cut himself and contract an infection in the workshop. 'But I don't want to sit in the house and worry. What good is that?'

I felt honoured to know a patient who lacked pretence. Ian had always had a generous spirit but now his wife noted a determination to craft some of his best woodwork as a way of saying goodbye. Ian's hobby was a metaphor for life: he would keep at it until he couldn't go on.

Dr Ranjana Srivastava

'Beyond thinking grateful thoughts, I need to do something with my hands,' he once laughed.

Signs of Ian's gratitude were everywhere. He regularly thanked the nurses for tolerating him even though he was their easiest patient. He commended the intern when she finally found a vein, and praised the secretary for fitting in a tricky appointment time. Everywhere I saw how he elevated a casual thank you to a high note and watched people beam at the recognition.

I could have had a transactional relationship with Ian and still done my job, but it was impossible not to be moved by his qualities. As various treatments stopped working, he would distract us both from feeling sad by asking about my children and their paintings, which adorn my office. He'd turn to parenting issues as if there were nothing more important on his mind. He talked proudly about his grandchildren, and when his daughter became tearful, eyes twinkling, he quipped, 'Well, life must be nearly complete if my oncologist knows all about the grandkids!' I laughed along but I also saw these remarks for what they were – endlessly innovative ways of paying tribute to the important people in his life.

Gratitude leavened his life. Without the means to look outward, anger, restlessness and discontentment may have crowded his twilight days. He might have kept asking 'Why me?' without receiving a satisfactory answer. Instead, gratitude was his tool of grace, his way of making the best of a bad situation. The result was a journey where he was held closely by everyone and was left in no doubt of the love and the legacy that would survive him. There could be no better dividend from his investment.

Keeping his word, Ian stopped chemotherapy when the bad days outweighed the good. He spent his last several weeks at home surrounded by his devoted family. He welcomed visitors and thrilled them with his spontaneous recollections of the fun they'd had together. Many were also consoled that they had made a difference.

Ian left school at a young age and always described himself as ordinary, but I think he was as enlightened a man as I had ever met.

After Ian's death, his family wanted to visit me, but I hastily reassured them that wasn't necessary. It can be trying for loved ones to visit a place associated with sad memories. But they all came and again I was struck by their poise, which pointed to how deliberately Ian had approached his death.

I told them how much I had learnt from Ian about living wisely and it meant a lot when they told me how fond he'd been of me. From her bag, his wife removed a hand-carved pen and handed it to me. 'Ian would have wanted you to have this.' I was touched but hesitated to accept something so precious. She insisted, saying he'd saved it for his final visit, which didn't eventuate. Knowing Ian, I believed that.

Dr Ranjana Srivastava

I toyed with keeping the gift in my office but on second thought, took it home to join the collection of objects and cards left behind by patients that remind me of the privilege of being a doctor.

Part 2

Conversations

*The art of conversation is the art of hearing
as well as of being heard.*

William Hazlitt

THE BEST PART OF MEDICINE is having meaningful conversations that allow people to make decisions that are in their best interest. Genuine conversation does not compete for the loudest voice or the strongest view but is an attempt to understand different perspectives. When we stop to listen, people become visible to us in all their complexity. We are all too used to walking the corridors of our own minds; conversations have the power to help us understand how others think. Ultimately, conversations bring us back to a better understanding of ourselves. They prompt us to define who we are and what really matters in our lives.

My whole work revolves around conversations. Doctors around the world complain that increasing administrative work is slashing the time actually spent with patients. Everyone knows that good conversations form the bedrock of meaningful decisions and the ones I have with patients nearing the end of life can be divided into three parts.

Early conversations necessarily focus on diagnosis and treatment. The ones in the middle are about helping people maximise their lives. The last have to do with dying well.

Not unlike our lives, the divisions aren't neat but they make for a useful framework.

An ancient Chinese proverb says that a single conversation with a wise person is the equivalent of a month's reading of books, but patients often protest that bookish knowledge is far easier to access than wise counsel.

There is tremendous pressure on doctors to know the answer to every illness. After all, this is the primary reason people consult us, to find out what's wrong with them. There would be fewer hit television dramas if doctors admitted the truth: many times, we aren't sure what to do and this is especially pertinent at the end of life.

In conversations about dying, an apprehensive doctor might say to a patient, 'Let me help you understand.' But it requires wisdom and maturity to ask the patient, 'Help me understand.' Experience has shown me that pretending to be an expert on mortality is to go on a fool's errand and it's far wiser to approach the task with humility and a willingness to learn from others.

This section of the book recounts some of the most important conversations that I have had with my patients at the end of life. Their stories illustrate the universal questions, dilemmas and practicalities people face.

Anyone who helps them navigate these issues understands how sensitive and difficult they are to ponder, but they are also essential in the quest to die well. Our conclusions may differ, but there is consolation in knowing that we are not alone in facing these challenges and there is wisdom in gleaning what we can from the lives of others

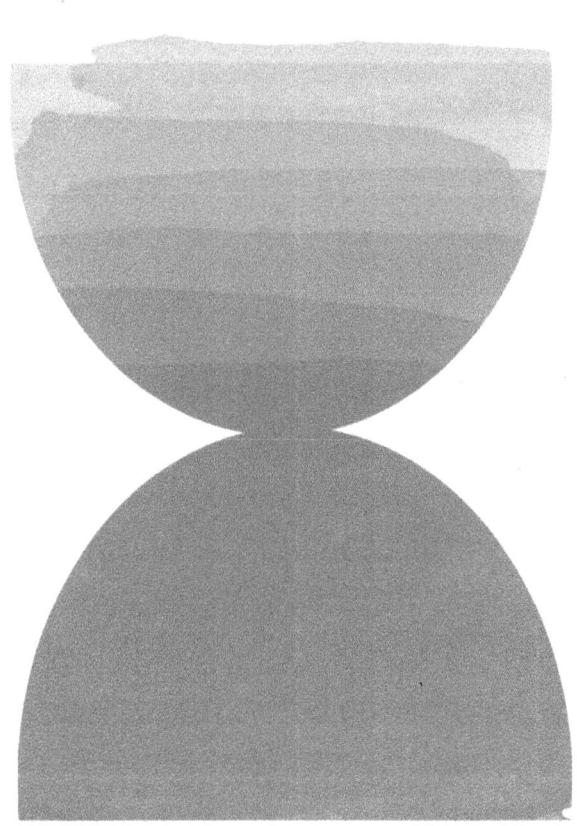

What doctors say, what patients hear

*The single biggest problem in communication
is the illusion that it has taken place.*
George Bernard Shaw

There are few things more upsetting to doctors than a terminally ill patient who says at the end of life, 'I had no idea.' I know it leaves me awash with questions about whether that patient might have made different decisions along the way had there been a greater appreciation of what an illness implied and an earlier acceptance of mortality.

But in an era where information rests at our fingertips, the idea of mortality is tucked far back in our minds. Studies show that most patients are unaware of a terminal prognosis and vastly overestimate their life expectancy. Sometimes patients are not told the facts, or they have misunderstood, but many people simply don't want to know.

In studies where cancer patients have been trained to ask questions about prognosis and end-of-life care, and their oncologists have consented to answering those questions frankly, the majority of patients choose to focus on more immediate issues such as the result of their blood test or the next line of treatment rather than a discussion about their preferences at the end of life. This might be human nature but not discussing mortality doesn't make it go away. It just robs us of the opportunity to decide how we live and how we die.

A lack of understanding about prognosis is responsible for causing immense emotional upheaval and hampering decision-making at the end of life. It is the single biggest reason for aggressive, expensive and futile medical interventions when it would be more appropriate and kinder to focus on supportive care. Precious days and weeks can be wasted like this, with the end result of universal dismay because the patient usually dies, the family is exhausted and the professionals are disillusioned.

Hilda was one of many patients I failed to convince of the limitations of medicine. She'd had worsening heart failure for three years and, by the time I met her, had developed such severe breathlessness and fluid retention that her equally elderly husband could no longer look after her. In hospital, the diuretics to offload excess fluid worsened her kidney failure and the cardiac medications dangerously lowered her blood pressure. She easily lost her balance and was deemed a high falls risk. Confined to bed, she became quickly deconditioned. This is the path of many chronic diseases but poor Hilda was flummoxed: why could no one fix her instead of just talking about things such as her kidneys or blood pressure that were invisible to her?

'What will you do for me?' she asked me every day. Unfortunately, I was doing all that I could. She could no longer keep up with the gradual deterioration in her health. This was the best septuagenarian she could be. Modern medicine hadn't failed her; in fact, it had helped her live as long as she had.

In this situation, it would have been best for Hilda to accept that further aggressive treatment would neither help her live longer or better. However, if the focus were to shift to quality of life, options such as oxygen, home help or residential care, something Hilda's husband wanted, could be explored. But Hilda was unmoved by my repeated requests for a frank conversation about her health. She scoffed at the notion that organ failure could result in the death of a patient who had survived breast cancer some thirty years earlier.

A proud and self-sufficient woman all her life, Hilda's denial came to define her and became her downfall. She spent a month in hospital without improvement. Then, annoyed by her perceived neglect, she discharged herself only to call an ambulance the next day to take her to a different hospital, where she languished from a hospital-acquired pneumonia. Her husband was near breaking point from driving to visit her every day and being asked to make decisions on her behalf when she became confused. Tragically, Hilda fell, fractured her hip and died. I was disheartened by how damaging a month of hospitalisation had been for her and how it had sapped her husband's energy. I kept thinking how different things might have been but for some tough conversations along the way.

But Hilda was far from alone; hospitals are full of patients who end up there through the revolving doors of modern medicine. Chronically ill and gravely deteriorating, they present to a hectic emergency department, which addresses their immediate problem but has neither the time nor the capacity to explore their expectations in detail.

Patients and relatives are asked what they want done but this is an unfair question when there is asymmetry of information between doctors and patients. Vulnerable patients reply they want 'everything done' because they're afraid their doctors will give up on them. But this reply only serves to trigger interventions about which questions are asked much later, often at mortality meetings where doctors and nurses wonder why no one suggested that doing nothing but providing comfort measures would have been the best option. No one I know is proud of this kind of medicine but it's what awaits us if we have never thought of ourselves as being mortal.

Nearly eighty per cent of people in developed countries wish to die at home surrounded by family and friends, but just ten per cent manage to have such a death. Sometimes practicalities prevent this but mostly people haven't thought ahead and run out of time to arrange the many logistics. Our lives will be to an extent unpredictable and the most careful preparation can still result in a fraught death, but many deaths would be better, and our loved ones spared the resulting trauma, if we took control.

This starts with being curious about our health. We should expect and demand better communication from professionals about diseases and their ramifications. But importantly, we must be willing to engage in conversations even when they test us. We must figure out how to broach the subject of dying and use the knowledge to live purposefully. Communication with professionals should be open and transparent and always let in a ray of hope. It should include trusted family members, recognising that they are the ones who help us carry our burden.

With foresight and preparedness, we can live meaningfully with the knowledge that death is universal and, when our day arrives, find ourselves prepared to face it.

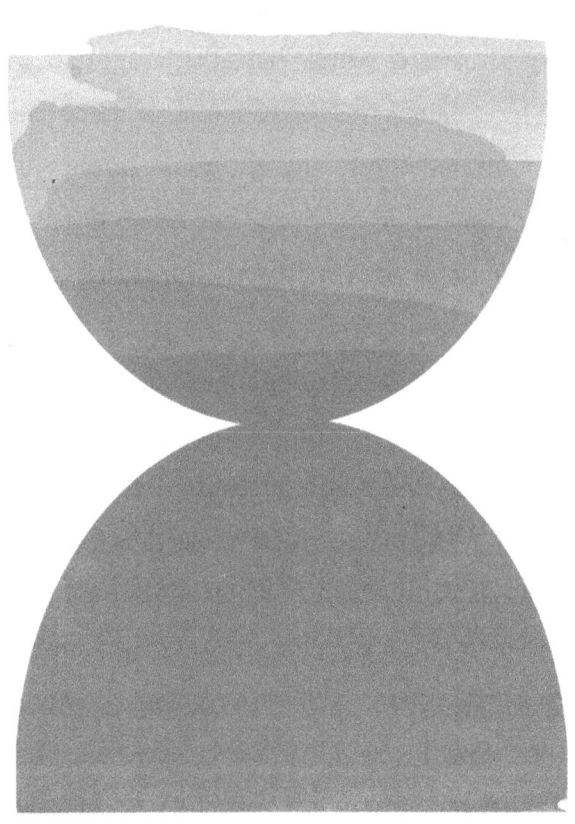

Giving patients the worst news

The truth is never pure and rarely simple.
Oscar Wilde

THE INTERPRETER GOT TO ME FIRST, with a face grown pale with concern. She whispered conspiratorially, 'Every time you say the word "cancer", the children want me to skip repeating it.' I sighed – all the seasoned interpreters were accustomed to such requests.

We would manage, I reassured the newcomer.

The children appeared more on edge than the patient, Yen, who sat in a wheelchair. Her forearm was plastered, a result of her latest fall on the way to the bathroom. Her rehabilitation was said to have been hampered by a diagnosis of cognitive impairment. Then she complained of abdominal pain and was unexpectedly diagnosed with cancer. I inferred from the notes that she didn't have long to live.

A discharge summary stated, 'In accordance with the family's request, cancer diagnosis not disclosed to patient.' I had to suppress my frustration.

No sooner did the family enter the room than the daughter made a beeline for me.

'We want you to tell Mum she has an ulcer.'

In my early years as an oncologist, my face would have revealed my incredulity. Now, I just said gently, 'She doesn't have an ulcer.'

'An infection then.'

I stayed quiet.

'People of her generation, they don't know any better,' she persisted. 'She doesn't know what any of it means but hearing "cancer" will kill her.'

Her claim sounded presumptuous, but it came from a place of love.

'Then it's my job to help her understand,' I gently replied.

Her brother stepped forward as I started to feel awkward at leaving Yen out of the conversation. 'In our culture, this is normal,' he insisted.

'I will understand if she doesn't want to know but I must give your mother the opportunity.'

'She has dementia, why burden her even more?' he reasoned.

I hated my predicament but had a duty of care towards Yen.

'If she has dementia, she won't understand me anyway, but at least I should try,' I negotiated.

He looked so downcast that I pledged to be kind as the interpreter wheeled the patient forward. The children closed in, as if poised to catch the grenade about to be lobbed.

'How are you?' I asked Yen.

'Quite well,' she replied via the interpreter. 'The arm hurts a bit but that's to be expected.'

From the way she answered my questions, her cognition seemed fine and I realised that pain and the language barrier must have made earlier assessment difficult.

'My inside hurts sometimes,' she offered when I asked about new symptoms. 'This is a new feeling.'

'Would you like to know why?' The children's gazes were on me, but I kept my eye on Yen.

She nodded eagerly. There was no doubt she wanted to know.

'You might remember having some scans. Unfortunately, they found cancer.'

'So, it *is* cancer? I thought so from the way everyone was acting.'

I couldn't help quietly celebrating her perceptiveness. Her children looked shocked, but she didn't bat an eyelid. Clearly, Yen had known all along but pretended otherwise because she wasn't supposed to know.

Giving patients the worst news

With a slight nod towards her children, she puzzled, 'But they said the scans were normal.'

'Mother, you must not worry,' her son exhorted. 'In our culture, we make peace with such things.'

She replied calmly, 'Of course we do, son.'

The tense outburst I'd feared never came; Yen's equanimity changed the tenor of the conversation.

Yen was a widow and the more I spoke to her, the more I realised she wasn't afraid to discuss her prognosis. This gave me the confidence to continue even though her children might have wanted me to stop.

'It would help me to know what you're thinking,' I said.

'I don't want to live forever, but I want to be home for as long as possible.'

I was touched by her simplicity. 'That's a goal we can work towards.'

I advised against further tests and contacted the palliative care team. She displayed her acumen again when she said her children might have questions they'd rather ask in her absence and offered to wait outside.

They explained that she'd nursed her ill husband at home with the help of palliative care, hence knew what to expect. This supported my view that people who have a positive experience of palliative care are more likely to welcome it in their own lives.

The children had many questions for me. We discussed the trajectory of her decline and how they should tell the rest of their traditional family. As we spoke, I could see them shed their internal guilt and conflict, their anxiety slowly replaced by confidence in handling what lay ahead.

A candid conversation about Yen's illness was very valuable. Like many patients I meet, Yen knew something was seriously wrong; full disclosure allowed her to plan ahead. For her children, it lifted an unenviable burden of concealing a serious diagnosis while caring for her increased needs. The family members and professionals she encountered were spared from practising deception, which never really works.

Later that day, the greatest surprise was a knock on my door.

'Doctor, I want to thank you for saving me,' the interpreter said after I had welcomed her into my office.

I was puzzled by her effusive praise until she explained. 'We belong to the same community, we pray together. I felt caught between loyalties although I always knew my job was to be *your* interpreter.'

Her words forced me to realise that the burden of withholding news of a terminal illness wasn't only carried by doctors and relatives but by unexpected others. Many relationships would have been tested by secrecy; however, Yen's knowledge and acceptance permitted people to grieve together and find mutual consolation. In her last days, Yen stayed calm, reiterating her wish to be kept free of pain. She told her children that her work on earth felt complete and expressed the hope of meeting her deceased husband in the afterlife.

Our conversation came full circle when her children later reflected that their experience had opened their eyes to a different way of handling death, although they confessed that traditional family attitudes would take time to change. I commended them, privately trusting that the memory of their mother's peaceful death would help them navigate the future.

The disclosure of a terminal diagnosis and the consequences of the disclosure are a live issue of debate in my work. In the 1960s, a staggering ninety per cent of oncologists admitted they would not disclose a terminal cancer diagnosis to a patient, believing that such knowledge would cause undue harm and detract patients from enjoying the twilight of their life. Just twenty years later, this view had become anachronistic and even insulting. Today, ninety per cent of oncologists say they would tell the patient. In an era of patient autonomy, full disclosure is seen as a moral, if not legal, obligation.

While I believe we all need to come to terms with our mortality, patients have a right to determine what and how much they want to know and we must always be mindful of cultural sensitivities.

Some people aren't ready for difficult conversations, but no patient who wants to know more should be neglected.

Doctors cannot be the sole arbiters of need, we must listen to our patients.

WORKING IN A DIVERSE COMMUNITY has shown me that everyone deals with death and dying differently. It's the norm in some cultures for family members to make important medical decisions on behalf of a patient. Some wives consider it a spousal duty that husbands should decide and I have encountered women who sought their husband's explicit permission to even talk to me. Sometimes, filial piety dictates that decisions are made by adult children, although I've been sad to see teenagers struggling to fulfil these roles too.

Withholding a terminal diagnosis can create medical, legal and, potentially, financial implications for the person being kept in the dark. But in other places, it's the norm for the patient to be the last to know – if they are told at all. Some cultures have a sincere belief that patients who can't change the outcome should be spared the worst news. It can be very confusing to know what to do.

Medicine emphasises the centrality of the patient, but a terminal illness creates a ripple in the whole family and, as I grow older, I have become more mindful of this. When I experience conflict between doing what I believe is right and bowing to the demands of the family, I have put the patient's best interest first. Since death is inevitable and irreversible, everyone deserves an opportunity to plan what remains of life, tie up loose ends and contemplate a legacy. This is what I say to people keen to shield their loved one from bad news and I am encouraged to find that this reasoning smooths out most objections.

Planning for the end of our lives does not need grand connotations. In fact, consolidating bank accounts, withdrawing superannuation funds, reducing a mortgage, using 'rainy day' savings, and – no small thing – putting together a list of passwords and authorisations are important for the dying patient as well as those grappling with the very modern task of achieving posthumous closure in a very practical sense. This has become a major hurdle for many survivors in an age of restricted access to personal information and I frequently meet families whose grief is magnified by a lack of organisation and planning on the part of the deceased. Spouses are bewildered by unmentioned loans, unpaid expenses and bankrupt businesses. Children have lost their education funds and elderly parents and relatives have suffered unanticipated loss and responsibility. The bitterness and resentment that arise from these real inconveniences are easily avoidable.

This is as good a place as any to mention the importance of making a will. In my experience, the absence of a will, an unclear or untraceable will causes some of the worst divisions in families. The potential for a problematic will to blast open minor cracks is confronting for onlookers, let alone those involved. In my career, some of the worst damage at the end of a patient's life has concerned a will. I have watched physical fights resulting in security incidents, brutal arguments at the bedside, and the closest of relatives vowing to never speak to each other again. My most disturbing memory is that of a family that demanded a dying patient's sedation be reversed so they could question his will. Of course, the staff refused but one can only begin to imagine the wounds of that family and wonder if they will ever recover.

In the emotion and reflection triggered by death, it is easier to misunderstand, misjudge and overreact but hostile words cannot be taken back. Sibling rivalry is a common cause of dispute, as are perceived inequality, suspected favouritism, a late marriage and the presence of stepchildren. Social workers recommend that, ideally, the discussion about a significant will takes place in the lifetime of the patient so that all parties are aware of wishes and instructions. The person making the will should ensure that it is accurate, current and stored with a trusted person. Much time is spent, and sorrow wasted, on tracing missing wills and pursuing intended benefits. The surprising thing is that it is often not the content of a will that loved ones fight over but the underlying principle. An essential part of dying well is to ensure that a will does not become a weapon. Again, this is made easier when we have understood our mortality.

Even if we have few personal effects, our business affairs are uncomplicated, and our will underwhelming, we all deserve the right to emotional closure. Mostly, the wishes of my patients feature reconciliation, forgiveness, taking holidays, writing letters, recording a legacy, and praying for strength and resolve. We should all give these matters the highest priority in a life well-lived. And while it's ideal to be more mindful of our priorities in our daily lives, the opportunity to make one final difference ought to receive the seriousness it deserves.

When it comes to discussing prognosis, it strikes me that we are not so much frightened of death as much as its prologue – that people will give up on us; there won't be any compassion, empathy or dialogue left. It should never be that way.

We will never know what people want and how they feel if we fail to ask. Assuming nothing and being open to everything comprises the art of medicine.

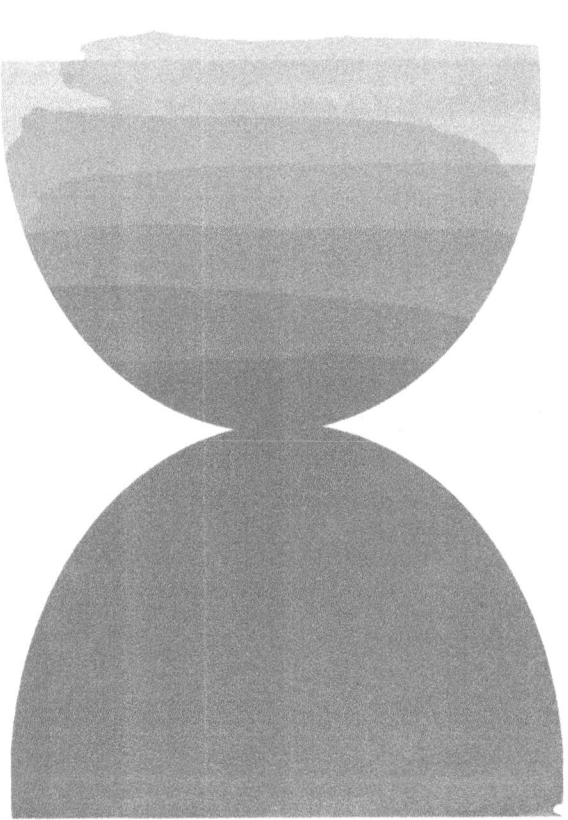

How people die

*While I thought I was learning how to live,
I have been learning how to die.*

Leonardo da Vinci

OUR CONSULTATION WAS NEARLY FINISHED when Richard leant forward.

'So, in all this time, no one has told me. How do people die?' Richard was eighty-three, with a crown of snowy hair and a face lined with experience. He had declined a second round of chemotherapy and entered palliative care. Curious at heart, he also wanted good explanations.

'What have you heard?' I asked.

'The usual stories.' He shrugged lightly but his concern was unmistakeable, and I suddenly felt protective of him.

'Should we discuss this today?' I asked gently, wondering if he might want his wife present.

'As you can see, I'm dying to know,' he replied, pleased at his own joke.

'How do people die?' is one of the most common questions cancer patients ask of Google. Cancer is just one of many conditions that lead to a gradual deterioration and death, so the explanation is relevant to anyone who has a chronic illness – from organ failure to dementia – that causes progressive decline.

While patients might google the answer, it's rare for them to ask their doctor. I have seen firsthand how the resulting fear and misconception can easily replace understanding when death approaches.

Some people are afraid to mention the subject, but others are firmly dissuaded from finding out more. 'When you mention dying, you stop fighting,' a man admonished his wife, but she suffered greatly for her lack of knowledge. Her religious family had kept her in the dark until days before her death she pleaded with me to tell her if she was dying.

'Yes, you are,' I said, holding her hand in mine. Her husband walked in just then and was furious at me for 'extinguishing her hope'. She apologised with her eyes while he hurled abuse at the staff and then, to our disbelief, discharged her from hospital. He refused palliative care services and insisted that my words had killed his wife. Incidents like this hurt the broader cause of communication at the end of life, but more importantly, they heap unnecessary trauma on the dying patient.

Many doctors feel reluctant to discuss prognosis because they can't be certain and it's also hard to convey bad news.

However, the evidence shows that sensitive and truthful conversation and, where appropriate, a discussion about mortality, enables patients to take charge of their healthcare decisions, plan their affairs and steer away from unnecessarily aggressive therapies.

It's natural to fear that an awareness of dying will increase suffering, and no one wants to make someone's dying days harder to bear. But it's worth emphasising that the evidence points to greater sadness, anxiety and depression when there is minimal awareness of dying.

Many of my patients describe short-lived unrest followed by tranquillity once their trepidation has been openly addressed. Where there is access, patients benefit greatly from palliative care professionals' support.

Not only is the dying process difficult for caregivers, but the burden also goes largely unrecognised. When people deteriorate over a number of years, prolonged stress causes carer exhaustion.

'I haven't slept well since Mum had her first stroke five years ago,' a patient's daughter said. 'It's a new normal.' Even when her mother was in respite, she felt the need to supervise timely medication and appropriate care.

Another carer who worked part-time to earn a living and cared for her terminally ill brother described the fear of losing him as a 'chokehold' on her life. She couldn't afford to compromise her job but felt guilty about leaving her brother with volunteers when she worked. She was determined to keep him home for as long as possible.

I saw in both cases how important it is for caregivers to be involved in conversations about declining health and expected death so that they are better equipped to deal with the dying process. How we experience the death of others also has a crucial bearing on how we deal with our own inevitable experience of death.

Not all diseases and not all patients behave the same. The human body is so complex and remarkable that to predict too much is to invite error, but none of this should stop us from understanding the process of dying. Death from cancer and many chronic diseases happens via what can be described as a common final pathway. 'Failure to thrive' is a broad term for the deterioration at the end of life.

Sufficient organ injury can lead to organ failure. Cancer is caused by an uninhibited growth of cells that expertly evade the body's usual defences to spread, or metastasise, to other parts of the body. Metastases to the liver, lungs, or brain eventually suppress vital organ functions causing death. Liver disease, heart failure or emphysema can occur due to habits like excessive alcohol intake, repeated heart attacks or prolonged smoking. The liver and kidneys, in particular, are responsible for eliminating toxins and maintaining normal physiology. Usually organs of great reserve, their failure is associated with death.

Chronic diseases including cancer result in the release of chemicals that suppress appetite and affect the digestion and absorption of food, leading to progressive weight loss. The interplay of these chemicals is poorly understood, and supplements don't seem to match the work of substances the body produces naturally. This is why appetite stimulants rarely work in sick patients and sleeping tablets don't reproduce the duration or quality of natural sleep.

As the body fails, dehydration can occur due to a distaste for fluids or an inability to swallow. The lack of nutrition, hydration and activity causes loss of muscle, weakness and fatigue.

Shortness of breath is a common feature of dying. Many cancer patients develop lung metastases. Heart and kidney failure result in fluid accumulation in the lungs. Severe emphysema depletes lung reserve. Consequently, many people can experience respiratory failure as 'air hunger', a feeling of not getting enough air to breathe.

Diseases such as cancer, diabetes and major organ failure impair immunity, making patients susceptible to infections. These infections can overwhelm the body's usual resources and treatment can be complicated by the difficulty of finding a safe antibiotic, especially in instances of liver or kidney failure. Fatal biochemical disturbances such as elevated potassium or calcium can occur due to underlying organ dysfunction.

Neurological conditions are a common cause of death. Brain metastases can result in severe fatigue, seizures, paralysis, bleeding and behavioural disturbance. Swelling of brain structures causes progressive loss of consciousness and death. Non-cancerous neurological conditions, in particular dementia, lead to debility via different means. Patients progressively lose critical aspects of brain function that maintain normal behaviour, impulses, appetite and bodily habits.

Essentially, our organs work in exquisite symphony and it's difficult to isolate the impact of one problem from the rest of the body.

The media commonly produces dramatised accounts of death, but contrary to popular belief, sudden and catastrophic death has become increasingly rare and the majority of deaths occur after predictable decline. This gives us an unprecedented opportunity to have a say in how we die.

It can be overwhelming to absorb all the details about how our bodies fail but modern medicine is slowly turning its attention to achieving a better death. The field of palliative care is important to this quest. Nurses, social workers, psychologists, pastoral care workers, and even pets play a vital role in ensuring that alleviating physical discomfort and psychological distress takes precedence over futile medical treatment.

Palliative care professionals are trained to tackle thorny questions, counsel patients and family members, and help them record a legacy. They normalise grief and reframe perspective. In areas where formal palliative care services are not available, it's useful to check for individual providers who have the same expertise.

It is sometimes feared that an introduction to palliative care is a replacement for effective medical care, but the evidence does not support this concern. Palliative care is not what happens when doctors have exhausted all other options. In fact, early introduction to palliative care while receiving active medical treatment has been shown to improve emotional health, quality of life and, in some cases, life expectancy, due to better attention to the whole person.

Many patients make more deliberate decisions when they understand their prognosis. Palliative care professionals help bridge the gap of understanding between doctors and patients, prompting the former to reflect on the value of continuing treatment and encouraging the latter to review their goals in life.

We have but one life and, as the end nears, we deserve an honest opinion, meaningful conversation, and compassion. Over 2000 years ago, the Greek philosopher Epicurus observed that the art of living well and the art of dying well were one. While we ought to be passionately interested in living well, we should care equally about dying well.

Dr Ranjana Srivastava

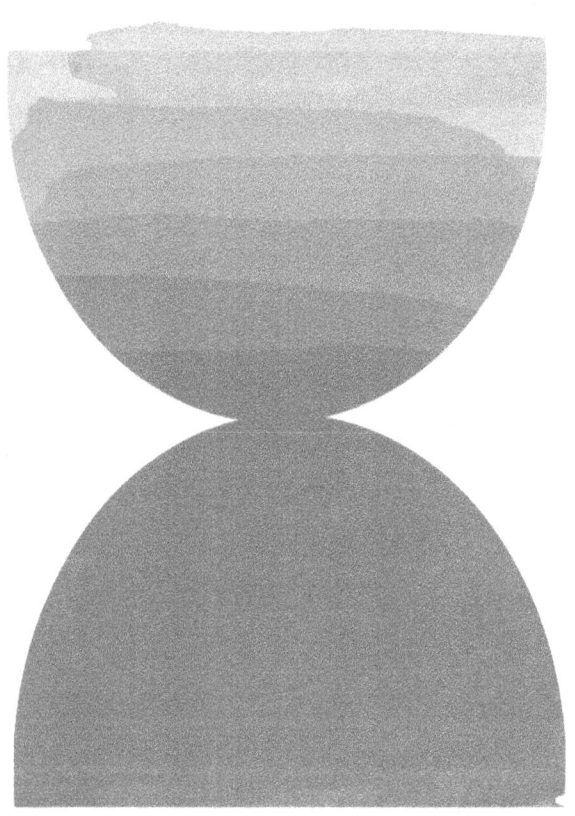

Deciding where to die

We're all just walking each other home.
Ram Dass

Everyone had a question for Zainab. Did it hurt? How much did it hurt? Was she drowsy? How bad was her nausea? Was she better or worse since the weekend? Those questions mattered but, when I met her, the most urgent question on my mind was where she wanted to die.

I hadn't met her before but her usual oncologist was away and there was no time to wait. I read that she had received cancer treatment for the past two years. Recently, a drug given as part of a clinical trial had triggered a serious reaction and now she was in hospital with a host of symptoms.

They had eased with medication but now she was very tired.

'I know things are bad,' she said quietly, after I'd introduced myself and asked how much she knew about her condition.

I quelled the temptation to gloss over this while thinking that one of the hardest conversations to have with strangers was about their mortality. But if we were to respect her end-of-life wishes, we needed to know them.

Zainab readily explained that she and her oncologist hadn't expected the clinical trial to provide much benefit, but they had both been surprised by how much worse it made her feel.

'Now I know I've tried everything,' she said. I noted that, rather than being disappointed, she sounded at peace. Meeting such patients is always a pleasure but the most evident benefit of equanimity in these circumstances is that it allows them to move beyond the present and plan for the future.

I knew I could ask Zainab this next question: 'If your health continued to fail, where would you like to be?'

'I'd love to be home,' she said thoughtfully. 'But I don't know if it's possible.' It can be hard to balance desire with practicality and many days can be wasted distinguishing between the two, but I thought Zainab would come to her own conclusion.

She told me she was widowed, retired and previously independent. In the last few months, she'd needed the support of her two sons and their families to continue to live alone. They had brought her nutritious food, taken care of her bills, and driven her to appointments. But now she needed more help, as there were days she didn't feel like getting out of bed or needed physical help in the shower. Zainab worried about falling but her main concern was for her sons. I was touched by her consideration.

'Have you thought about alternatives to home?' I asked.

'That depends on how long I have to live,' she replied matter-of-factly, and again I was struck by her clarity of thought.

No one likes to deliver bad news but this was a time that demanded the truth.

'I'm sorry to say, weeks.'

'Yes, that's what I thought,' Zainab nodded, absolutely unbowed, as if we were discussing a delivery date for furniture. Her resilience was stunning; I sensed it arose from a place of contemplation and acceptance.

'I'll accept hospice but I'd like to explore going home.' She doubted that her sons could help as they'd found it confronting watching their grandmother grow thin and frail before she died but agreed with the social worker that they should be involved in the decision.

Zainab's prediction proved accurate. Her elder son was anxious and spoke very little. It was immediately obvious that he would not cope with his mother dying at home. The younger son confessed that, much as he'd like to, he didn't think he could give his mother the care she deserved.

The social worker reassured them that many families felt the same. At the same time, I was bitterly disappointed for Zainab. Part of me wished we'd never called the meeting with her sons. But Zainab surprised me yet again by praising her sons for their willingness to be involved and acknowledging the sadness of tending the dying. Deftly, she had moved to preserve sibling harmony after her death.

Later, she told me that since she had not expected them to care for her, she didn't feel let down. The social worker thought Zainab was one of the most stoic and measured patients she had ever met. In fact, her conduct fostered so much goodwill that her sons joined forces with some neighbours and took her home for day visits and a surprise garden party that thrilled her.

When a hospice bed became available, Zainab went there to spend the last ten days of her life, dying faster than I had predicted. She was very grateful for the nursing care as well as the constant presence of her sons. Zainab's ability to handle the truth, ask questions without fear and adjust her expectations played a large role in dying well.

The question of where to die has become a modern-day dilemma. A recent survey in the UK showed that although only one per cent of cancer patients express a preference to die in hospital, more than a third do. Overall, only twenty per cent of all patients in western countries manage to die at home. Indeed, the prevalence of hospitalised dying led a newspaper headline to protest that thousands of patients were being 'denied' their wish to die at home. I thought this headline disregarded the complex nuances of end-of-life care while unintentionally heaping guilt on exhausted caregivers.

Many people express an intention to die at home at a time when they are still able to manage, albeit with increasing difficulty and help from dedicated relatives. Commonly, their health worsens, their relatives can provide limited assistance, external providers can only fill some of the gap and, suddenly, remaining at home becomes impractical or unsafe.

Being home is a visceral need for many and health professionals devote themselves to making it happen, but when once-simple activities like turning in bed, taking medications safely or fixing lunch become a challenge, the only way to get home is with round-the-clock care, which is unaffordable for the majority of people.

If it takes a village to raise a child, it also takes one to help someone die at home.

A dying patient requires a constant, if not continuous, presence of carers who are physically robust and have the emotional resilience to withstand the ups and downs of the dying process. There is no doubt that, even for the most prepared, this work is exhausting. The days are long and filled with concern about whether there is a right way of doing things. In a society not used to inter-generational care taking place at home, it can be anxiety-provoking for those thrust into this role. Add to this the unpredictability of how long end-of-life care may last and the challenge grows. But many loved ones wouldn't have it any other way for they know they bring solace to the dying and consider their work significant and life-affirming.

People with similar diagnoses can have a very different illness trajectory. A weary carer recently reflected that she had been waiting for eight months for her mother to die from a stroke that was meant to have killed her within eight hours. The daughter of a dementia patient felt sorely for her father, who contracted infections that he kept surviving despite not being given antibiotics. One of my cancer patients survived longer than the few months she had been expected to live, which plunged her barely managing husband into depression. I will never forget the case of a cognitively impaired patient on dialysis whose elderly and overwrought wife attempted suicide because she couldn't see another way out. In all cases, family members were deeply conflicted about wanting a loved one to die rather than suffer from poor quality of life.

Caregivers are some of the most unappreciated people in society. They brace themselves for physically hard and emotionally gruelling work, often relinquishing other priorities such as their job, social life and even their own health. The idea of duty sustains them.

Dr Ranjana Srivastava

It goes without saying that there are many people who would like to do these things but simply can't. As the population ages, many caregivers are themselves elderly, frail or ill. Frequently, my elderly dying patients are the primary carer for an elderly spouse or a disabled adult child.

Sometimes, adult children who have fallen on hard times move back with a parent. Sometimes the arrangement is mutually beneficial and allows a terminally ill person to remain at home but, depending on circumstances, it can also add enormous stress. The growing problem of alcohol and substance abuse has left more than a few of my terminally ill patients caring for young grandchildren and navigating the legal system to secure their future. I've met children as young as ten providing care for a seriously ill parent, but it would be impossible to expect that child to manage end-of-life care. These are all people who cannot do any more than they already are.

We must acknowledge the discomfort and fear involved in caring for the dying. In a mobile society, we have also become removed from the day-to-day lives of our loved ones, making it difficult to provide intimate care.

By housing our ill, disabled and elderly in institutions, we let strangers perform the difficult task of caring for them. While modern life might make it necessary to enlist help from institutions, Australian research shows that nearly half of nursing home residents receive no visitors. Loneliness, malnourishment, and emotional deprivation are common.

Providing end-of-life care at home may not be for everyone but contemplating our own end of life must be. A society that doesn't think about mortality struggles to know what to do when faced with the dying. We don't just place our elderly and vulnerable in homes; we forget about them. Their deterioration makes us uncomfortable and their death reminds us of our own future selves. We end up avoiding the essential truth of our own mortality.

There's a widespread sense that death has become too medicalised. It's true that even a short stint in hospital spells noise and disruption. It's hard to get sleep and impossible to find a comfortable bed or a hot cup of tea. But amid all this, hospitals do provide – and patients appreciate – clinical expertise. There are caring nurses, vigilant doctors, continuous supervision and proper symptom relief. Social workers and chaplains impart calm confidence in the face of challenges. Psychologists address grief and volunteers offer company.

Anyone who has cared for the dying knows that alleviating existential distress is as important as securing physical comfort. Institutions manage symptoms better than emotions, but many carers confess to being so exhausted meeting a patient's daily needs that tapping into grief can seem like a luxury.

When institutions step in to assume the physical burden, dealing with the emotion of dying seems more possible.

Of course, hospitals are imperfect and make some awful blunders, but we shouldn't underestimate the comfort they bring to dying patients and their loved ones. An increasingly common request from my dying patients relates to staying longer in a hospital or going to hospice. We cannot dismiss the fact that there are many people at the end of life who feel safe there.

The question is not whether dying patients need professional support but what form it should take. Robust community palliative care and greater availability of inpatient hospice are the obvious alternatives to acute hospitals. Evidence shows that palliative care is beneficial and cost-effective but, despite this, it's inadequately funded, sometimes misunderstood, and frequently overstretched. For palliative care to fulfil its mission, patients must be confident that it will be available when they need it. Symptoms at the end of life can change quickly and a week-long delay in response can seem like a lifetime. A good relationship with a family doctor who is available to provide end-of-life care and counsel also has a great impact on the decision to go home.

Discussions about where to die are onerous for professionals and patients. After twenty years of experience, I know I still struggle with them. But if we want to do our best, doctors must be bold enough to broach the subject of dying and patients and loved ones must find the courage to engage. The experience of caring for a dying patient leaves an unforgettable mark on caregivers and determines how they view their own mortality. Hence, there's a dual benefit to approaching the subject thoughtfully.

For most of us, where we die is less important than how we die. We can ease the experience by understanding the limitations of curative medicine and recognising that the other great job of modern medicine lies in offering peace to the dying and solace to survivors.

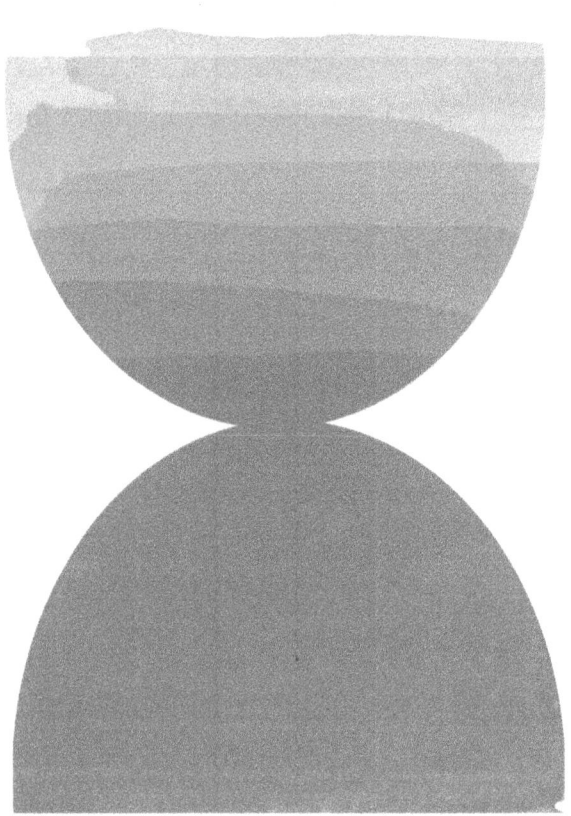

Getting the best care at the end of life

*If a man knows not to which port he sails,
no wind is favourable.*

Seneca

For centuries, medicine had nothing more to offer than balms, potions and the healing touch of a physician. The philosopher Voltaire rightly remarked that the art of medicine consists of amusing the patient while nature cures the disease. A century of progress has transformed medicine unrecognisably. We are living well longer, diseases once deemed a death sentence have been controlled or eradicated, and ordinary people have greater access to information. Doctors are armed with better evidence, smarter drugs and more accurate technology. But few would argue that medicine still has a long way to go towards responding to the needs and preferences of the patient as a human being.

A recent Australian study found that 41,000 days in hospital every year – amounting to an annual cost of over 150 million dollars – were devoted to what a range of specialists deemed to be non-beneficial care at the end of life, resulting in an average of fifteen days each patient spends in hospital and five days in intensive care. Futile treatment at the end of life is a common occurrence in many countries. In the United States, it's estimated that five per cent of the population accounts for fifty per cent of the cost of healthcare and while the exact figures may vary, the point is that for most people living in developed countries, healthcare spending will be increasingly concentrated in the final weeks of life. And while the definition of futility is subjective, and economic truths are hard to reconcile with emotional decisions, the truth is that patients at the end of life are highly vulnerable, the decisions they are asked to make are very complex, and it's tempting for everyone to fall into the trap of believing that more is better.

Thirty thousand scientific journals publish over a million scientific papers every year, mostly celebrating positive studies that push another drug or intervention to the market. Only a small fraction of these studies are actually life-changing, but since it is impossible to keep up with the data, doctors mostly rely on a few experts and the pharmaceutical industry to interpret the findings. Bias, conflicts of interest and selective publishing abound in medicine. Drug companies have a vested interest in promoting the benefits, but not the risks, of drugs. Opinion leaders in medicine are frequently found to be guilty of research and publishing misconduct. These concerns go unnoticed by the general public and can appear tedious to the wider medical profession, which wants easily digestible information to treat growing numbers of patients. Consequently, it's not hard to see how hype transcends reason.

I am often asked about the greatest challenge in medicine. I daresay it is to empower people to have an important say in how they die. It has never been more important to ensure that proposed medical interventions are thoughtful, considered and compatible with their goals of care. Needless to say, this demands a rethink of the prevailing culture; we simply cannot make decisions about dying well without accepting our mortality.

⁂

AT NINETY-FIVE, MY PATIENT HAROLD wanted only one thing: a hot cup of tea. Since his wife died, he'd been managing alone, content with sitting in his favourite armchair and sipping his tea with the radio for company. His children kept pressing him into residential care, but he wouldn't hear of it. One day, his daughter found him slumped in his chair after suffering a stroke. He was brought to hospital, where all his family agreed that he should be allowed to die peacefully.

But Harold didn't die; instead, he came to my medical ward in a semi-conscious state.

Thanks to evidence-based care, the outcomes for stroke patients have greatly improved. Early interventions are credited with saving lives and improving quality, but any evidence must be tailored to the needs of the individual. Protocols were never meant to be applied indiscriminately.

Harold was disabled by his stroke. His weak side prevented him from sitting in a chair so he was mostly propped up in bed, where he intermittently dozed. His speech and swallowing were altered but there was one thing he told anyone who would listen: he was desperate for a cup of tea.

Passersby would sympathise before pointing to the sign above his bed warning he was at risk of aspiration, which means food or drink entering the airway instead of the stomach due to the swallowing mechanism being impaired. Aspiration can cause pneumonia, a common cause of hospitalisation and death in the elderly.

Following the stroke protocol, the speech pathologist had tested Harold and pronounced him fit for only artificially thickened drinks and pureed foods, both of which he intensely disliked. If he wanted water, it had to be mixed with a thickener, but as anyone who has tasted thickened water knows, it's no match for the refreshing taste of normal water. Poor Harold tried it and spat it out.

Most reasonable people would suggest that a man in his mid-nineties should be allowed to eat and drink as he pleased, even if aspiration resulted in pneumonia or death. A cup of tea is certainly what I wanted for Harold, but I had scarcely expected the commotion this would cause.

When patients are mostly asleep or aren't able to express themselves fully, an assumption is made that their cognition isn't intact and that decisions about their care need to be made by others. The speech pathologist advised Harold's children about the danger of drinking tea and they immediately balked at the thought that, after surviving a stroke, their father could die from aspiration. The children admonished Harold not to have tea and he was mostly too tired to argue. I saw that his prognosis was poor regardless of what else happened and eventually convinced the speech pathologist of the bigger picture. But now, it was difficult for the family to budge from its position. Two of his children were sympathetic but the other two were determined to avoid any risk to Harold.

The impasse continued all week before the social worker called a meeting to find a solution.

I had to use my best persuasive powers to convince the family that to allow Harold to have his cup of tea actually constituted good medical care. That day, Harold was wide awake to firmly state what he wanted, and I felt quietly triumphant when the meals attendant whispered how happy she was to have served him what he hankered for. Finally, Harold got his cup of tea. He didn't live happily ever after but the few months he lived were made more bearable by cups of tea.

To an outsider, it might seem preposterous that the thorniest dilemma in the care of a frail old man was whether or not to let him have a cup of tea, but Harold's story was a case in point that the biggest impact can be made by heeding the smallest desires of patients.

It should be possible to benefit from the best of what medicine has to offer without being a victim of all that it can do, and for this, we must be active participants in our care. We must believe that we won't live forever, but as long as we live, we will do so in a meaningful way. When we cannot speak for ourselves, we need our loved ones to be our confident advocates, bold enough to distinguish between what we want and what they think we should want.

It is vital that doctors pause their frantic activity and ask what matters to patients. All too often, medicine takes on an energy of its own that loses sight of the patient. In turn, this places a great responsibility on patients to insist on being a part of the conversation about what's happening to them.

I'm frequently moved to see how my dying patients vex over all kinds of decisions and often get hopelessly lost in the minutiae. Wondering about whether or not to have more treatment, undergo more tests and seek further opinions at the end of life can overwhelm even the most resilient individual but my advice to patients has always been that each decision point comes back to what really matters to them. The answer is different for us all but those who can answer the big questions always manage to find the answers to the smaller ones. The German philosopher Nietzsche put it best when he observed that 'He who has a why to live for can bear almost any how.'

For Harold, who had led a full life, and greatly missed his wife's company, happiness meant a cup of tea. For some of us, it might mean going fishing, holding a grandchild, or celebrating one last birthday in style. For others, there's deep satisfaction to be found in recalling their legacy, sitting in their garden or caressing a pet. When compared to the sophistications of modern medicine, these needs sound simple and unpretentious, but these are the things we ought to take seriously because they form the bedrock of a meaningful life.

When we look around, many of us feel worried about the mismatch between what patients want and what doctors do, but it is possible to receive the best of what medicine has to offer by thinking about our goals in life.

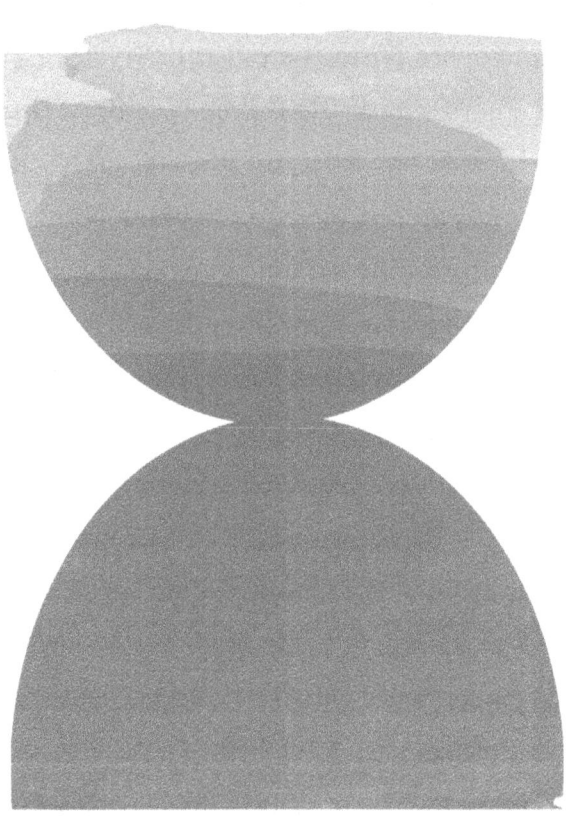

Letting go

*It is not death that a man should fear
but he should fear never beginning to live.*

Marcus Aurelius

THE PATIENT'S SCREAMS reverberated around the intensive care unit until it was hard to fathom how such suffering could exist within the walls of a sophisticated hospital. It was impossible to focus amid the commotion and the many pained expressions that greeted it.

I found out from a nurse that a frail, bed-bound woman with dementia had developed a gangrenous foot. Her family had initially decided against an amputation, as recovery would be impossible, but when her consciousness began to falter due to sepsis, so did their determination to avoid an operation.

The family now decided that the patient should undergo

surgery despite the risk. This is a common enough situation and it's possible that sitting down with the family and absolving them of the responsibility they felt for her impending death would have allowed the patient to die peacefully. This required an explanation that there was more at stake than surviving the surgery itself, there also needed to be some measurable benefit to a cognitively impaired patient. But these negotiations take time and, faced with a deteriorating patient and an insistent family, the decision was made to amputate the septic foot and hope for the best.

The patient survived the surgery but never recovered the little function she'd had. A month later, she remained confused, visibly distressed and unable to communicate. Her background dementia worsened as a result. The intensive care unit was pierced by her cries until she was sent to the ward, where she spent another few months because the family could no longer manage her care. When she finally went home, it was with costly community supports, round-the-clock family attendance, and no insight into her situation.

For all those who met her, this poor woman was a stark representation of the lingering death we all fear, and her case prompted much soul-searching. She symbolised the worst of what happens when we are incapacitated, have not made our wishes clear beforehand, and our loved ones are hard-pressed to decide what is in our best interest.

Dr Ranjana Srivastava

Watching her prolonged suffering, I couldn't help thinking back to patients and families who had succeeded in letting go when it mustn't have been easy. The most memorable of such patients was Ali.

At just twenty-two, Ali packed in the poise and wisdom of someone thrice his age. He had arrived in hospital with abdominal pain thought to be appendicitis but emerged from surgery with a diagnosis of advanced cancer. Everyone was devastated. The surgeon, with children of her own, was clearly shaken when she told him and his parents that she could not offer a cure.

I had dreaded my first meeting with them because I rarely looked after patients as young as Ali. I didn't know what I could say to console them but I wanted to be truthful. I said that I, along with everyone, was saddened and puzzled by Ali's diagnosis. His illness was incurable, but I would dedicate myself to helping him live as long as possible. Ali was understandably overwhelmed and quiet while his parents had many questions, which they asked calmly and sensitively. I thought how fortunate he was to have their support.

Ali began chemotherapy but unfortunately kept running into complications that put him in hospital. After his third admission in seven months, he suggested a family meeting attended by his parents and twin sisters, which I convened with considerable trepidation. I invited a pastoral care worker and a palliative care nurse to the meeting, glad that doctors have able people to help them have difficult conversations if they only ask.

Ali was supposed to be at university, tackling things not much harder than what subjects to study and how many hours to work at his local library; instead, he was confronting the prospect of dying. How did someone so young reconcile to his fate while his grandparents were still playing golf? How could he fairly look back at his life and say he'd had enough?

As I would discover, Ali had been reading, talking and thinking about his illness and its implications all along. I watched in admiration as he capably took charge, acknowledging that the circumstances were grim, but everyone needed to talk openly.

He told us that he didn't want further treatment for his terminal illness because it impacted his quality of life. He felt sad at missing out on future experiences with his family but was eager to make the most of his time. He believed that time well spent would reduce his regret and leave his family good memories to cherish. Some things he wanted to do included a fishing trip with his dad, a karaoke party with his siblings, and baking his favourite cake with his mother.

Until then, I had been to hundreds of meetings but had seldom seen one where I needed to do nothing except sit back and reflect on the impossible courage and equanimity of a young man. I know that the other professionals were also holding back their tears.

I had been dreading the mood in the meeting. It would have been tragic to see an outpouring of grief or, worse, conflict about the direction of care. But the way Ali spoke, with care and conviction, actually lifted the heavy mood and succeeded in energising his whole family to help him achieve what he wanted.

No one tried to dissuade him; instead, the focus shifted immediately and excitedly to getting him out of hospital to do what he wanted. It was a beautiful thing to be a part of the concerted effort to make Ali's last days count. His acceptance made it easier to have frank conversations with him and allowed a string of professionals to express their admiration for him and say goodbye.

Ali went home with palliative care and his mother kept in touch with the hospital. I learnt that he fulfilled his first list of wishes and moved on to a second. Not having treatment spared him its toxicity and, as he often reminded his family, allowed him to be home, the place he loved the most.

The palliative care team was invaluable in providing pastoral support and buoying the family's spirits by praising their dedication to Ali. Ali's family doctor had known him since he was a child – she too swallowed her sadness and dedicated herself towards helping him.

Ali's mother reflected that, while no parent imagined losing a child, what really struck her was the family's ability to persevere through its pain.

There were times, she said, when they were together as a family and forgot that Ali was dying. I was curious to know how this was possible when many grieving families struggled to maintain a semblance of normality in the face of death. She acknowledged that from time to time it was inevitable that they talked about events that Ali would not see, including the twins graduating, his parents' golden wedding anniversary or the next family reunion, but mostly, they savoured the present.

She observed that the family worked hard at being stoic, mentioning their devastation coupled with the determination that Ali would die on a positive note. Her words felt like a weight on my heart because they renewed my regret, but I felt privileged to see that people of any age could work towards a better death.

Thanks to his attitude and the family's help, Ali enjoyed his life for a few months before declining over two weeks. As he grew weaker, the activity around him slowed. Visitors were politely limited, and the family closed ranks. They kept a quiet vigil at his bedside, spoke softly and moved gently. Ali and his family were brave to the end, reminding each other to be grateful for their time together.

Dr Ranjana Srivastava

We are not born with a rulebook for letting go but Ali's family learnt how. The family sat with him as he breathed his last. They had always known that his death would leave a hole in their lives and they worked through his death as through his life, with unity, forbearance and love.

Not long after Ali died, I came upon a Buddhist quote that summed up perfectly my unforgettable experience of knowing him and his family. 'In the end only three things matter: how much you loved, how gently you lived, and how gracefully you let go of things not meant for you.'

Part 3

Advice for patients and their families

For it is in giving that we receive.
Francis of Assisi

DOCTORS ENTER MEDICINE with the aim of making a difference, and understand the need to provide holistic care, but can be let down by the constantly whirring wheels of medicine. Something that hampers my ability to care for patients is the amount of paperwork and authorisations required. While adequate documentation is necessary, the problem arises when it takes precedence over actual care. There is no substitute for talking to patients and understanding their circumstances and motivations, and a growing frustration among many health professionals is that the time to do this is lost to filling out forms to satisfy bureaucratic demands.

This problem is particularly pointed at the end of life in an institutional setting, commonly a hospital or residential care, where eighty per cent of patients die. The most important aspect of caring for the dying is to administer care and comfort and provide physical touch and emotional sustenance but even in this phase of life, the notes, forms and checklists leave surprisingly little time for the patient and even less for families. All this makes dying much less of the communal event it once was and underlines the loneliness of the experience.

For those in hospital, the changing guard of doctors and nurses is overwhelming. The average patient can expect to meet dozens of different professionals without a clear idea of who they are and what role they have. People who die at home have a variable experience depending on the availability of practical help and professional expertise. Even the most prepared patients and the most motivated families need help to navigate one of the most challenging periods in their lives.

My experience of caring for the terminally ill has attuned me to the disempowerment of patients and loved ones. They are particularly afraid of getting things wrong. Are they strong enough advocates? How can the whole family survive the process? Is it okay to grieve? What should they ask friends to do?

Years of such conversations have illuminated my understanding and shown me that learning from others can give us all the confidence to help the dying.

The following section contains advice for patients and families on how to help each other in the quest for a better death.

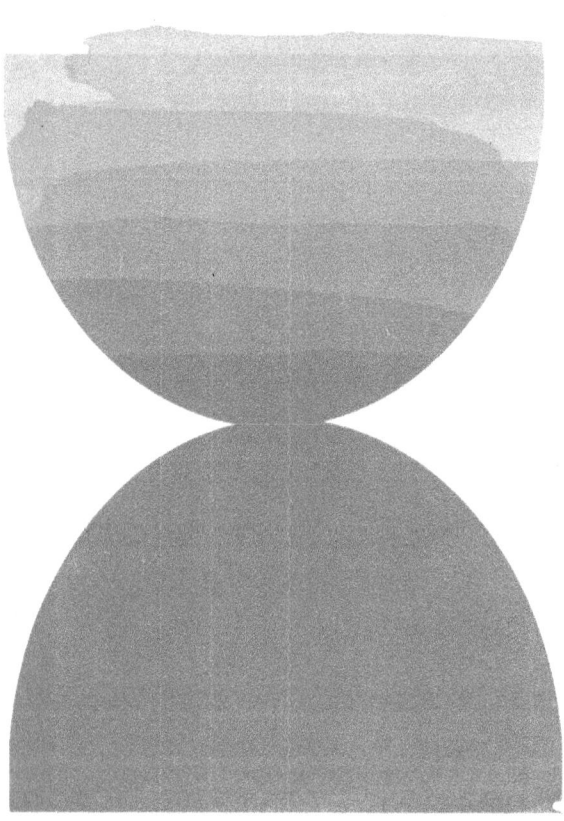

Handling conflict within families

*If you want to change the world,
go home and love your family.*

Mother Teresa

JOSIP AND MARTA had been married for fifty of their seventy years. They met at age five and couldn't remember a time without each other. Together, they had a son but Marta's pregnancy was so complicated that she was unable to have the brood she desired. But their son was wonderful and all that they had hoped for.

In the same month as she retired from her teaching job, Marta became my patient. She hadn't been well for a few weeks but when her breathing grew more difficult, she came to hospital. She was sent home but soon returned feeling worse. This time, she was diagnosed with advanced cancer and admitted to the ward, where I was scheduled to meet her the following day. But a concerned intern urged I should see her sooner.

That evening, I found Marta lying in bed looking very tired. Her laboured breathing was making her pale and clammy. She hadn't eaten or slept in a few days and my first thought was that she might die during the night. Making a mental note to commend the intern, I set about making Marta comfortable with the help of an insightful nurse. Together we set up a morphine infusion and watched Marta relax as the drug took effect. But before going home, I had the heart-wrenching job of telling Marta and Josip that she might not have long to live. Marta nodded, too ill to speak. A downcast Josip pleaded with me to do my best. I sensed their unspoken question about whether her care had been delayed and truthfully told them that, while an accurate diagnosis two weeks ago would have been psychologically beneficial, it would not have altered her survival. I know how much the question gnaws at families long after a patient dies.

After forty-eight hours, Marta turned the corner. Morphine eased her breathing and she was able to speak although she was still precariously ill and not fit to receive any treatment beyond supportive measures.

In an era where modern drugs and technology keep some patients alive for years, it can be baffling for others to hear that they aren't suitable for any treatment. But Marta had appraised her situation and concluded that she was dying and too weak to go home.

In the following days I noticed that Josip kept a constant vigil at his wife's bedside and only went home to shower and change. Nights of sleeping in a hard chair were taking their toll on him and I became concerned at his increasingly worn look. Bad news sometimes leads to a string of visitors; I saw a few of Marta's friends but never met her son, who I kept expecting to have many questions on behalf of his quiet parents.

'He should come some time,' Josip said tentatively as Marta dozed. I caught the strain in his voice.

That weekend, I slipped in to see Marta to see if her morphine infusion needed adjusting to reach a balance between symptom relief and sedation. I was gratified to hear that she felt comfortable and well cared for. Josip, meanwhile, looked haggard and sheepishly admitted to surviving on canned food.

His remark piqued my curiosity about his son's support but I didn't want to pry. Perhaps Josip was at the end of his tether because the next question he asked was whether he could see a psychologist. His request caught me by surprise, and I told him that I could call for a chaplain, but he'd need to see his family doctor for more help.

'Everyone has been so good to us,' he said.

'That's because you're easy to care for,' the nurse just entering the room smiled.

Her remark broke his reserve. With tears flowing freely, he took out a folded letter from his wallet, handing it to me. My eyes widened as I read a stinging diatribe from the son, criticising Josip for neglecting Marta and 'putting on a show' in hospital. The son professed his hatred for his father, squarely blaming him for the unfolding tragedy of his mother's death. The vitriol contained in the letter left me aghast.

As I read the letter, Josip wept with shame.

Half-awake now, Marta reached out for his hand. 'He is angry and doesn't know what to do.' Overcome with emotion, she stopped but the nurse and I sensed he had more to say.

We heard about the son's marriage breakdown and his subsequent mistrust of close relationships and descent into substance abuse. He had reacted poorly to the news about his mother and couldn't bear to visit her in hospital. Since the diagnosis, father and son hadn't spoken and Josip revealed he was afraid of repercussions when Marta died.

I held the letter limply in my hands, wishing Josip would tear it up. All too often, I'd seen the conflict unleashed through unguarded speech. As Marta lay dying, the son's words had caused the kind of pain that no medicine could reverse.

Marta was deeply hurt by her son's actions but recognised that she didn't have time to help him, and was determined that he remember her as a mother who loved him till the end. Marta deteriorated rapidly and in her final days made the monumental decision to not see her son at all, wanting only Josip by her side.

I could scarcely imagine the wound in her heart. It was saddening for Marta to be deprived of the closure she deserved and for Josip and his son to have lost the opportunity for reconciliation. But people with close knowledge of the situation thought that Marta had acted wisely.

Josip and I talked at length about the grief, regret and myriad other emotions experienced by loved ones when someone is dying. These emotions are complex, intense and unpredictable. We often aim to shield our children but for adults, too, the turmoil can be deeply unsettling.

My work exposes me to the best and the worst of grieving families. I have learnt that in all but the rarest of instances there is hope for reconciliation, but it starts with an essential belief that we have a finite time to address the ties that matter to us. I've witnessed the transformative effect of a phone call, a hug or an apology, and I've seen a heartfelt letter or the smallest gift change the dynamic. It's okay to take the step that feels the safest.

Some of the best people to help start an important conversation when time is short are chaplains, social workers and counsellors and I strongly recommend their services to families. The difficulty of finding reconciliation should never dissuade us from taking the first steps.

While it's common to feel helpless as we decline, there are some things that we can control.

A family meeting is a good way to address issues that are important to multiple people so that everyone hears the same message. An objective person such as a friend or a professional can be asked to facilitate such a meeting to ensure it adheres to its purpose.

Something that causes tremendous upheaval in even close families is disagreement over the direction of care of a dying parent. Some relatives can accommodate mild differences but strongly opposing views and ideological differences can quickly derail good end-of-life care. The alternatives of involving a legal professional or seeking state guardianship are time-consuming and often impractical; in reality, when significant stakeholders can't agree, medicine errs on the side of continuing to do more until there is consensus.

One way to avoid this is by creating an advance care directive, sometimes referred to as a living will. Our recorded instructions and wishes would have our personal authority and the legal recognition to end most disagreements. People worry that an advance care directive may not be respected by professionals — and it's prudent to ensure your directive is correctly written and witnessed – but I hasten to point out that the real issue is that the vast majority of people have never thought about their death and never documented their wishes. Professionals increasingly welcome insight into the patient's wishes and make every attempt to honour them. So, if we have ever thought about the kind of medical fate we'd like to avoid, for instance prolonged intensive care unit admission, futile resuscitation attempts, artificial nutrition or other unacceptable interventions, we must take the next step of making them known.

A less formal alternative to a living will is appointing a surrogate decision-maker to articulate our wishes when we are unable to do so. But this means letting them know clearly what we want. It's not possible and also very onerous for someone to guess at our intimate thoughts about dying and make critical decisions on our behalf.

Dying well involves looking after ourselves but also being mindful of our loved ones.

I LOST MY GRANDMOTHER when I was young. My conversations with my *nanima* never made it beyond what delicious fare she could cook for me and when I would visit her again. When I last saw her, I didn't fully understand what a last visit meant but I could feel the emotion in the air wrap itself around me.

Now that I'm a parent and my mother is a grandparent, I can begin to calculate the heartache in the room. My *nanima* wordlessly pressed two small gold beads into my hands, which my mother later had made into earrings. More than thirty years later, they are somewhat bent but still shiny. I regard them with a fondness that I have for few other possessions and look forward to passing them on to my daughter. The earrings are a physical reminder of my history and a tribute to my grandmother, who would have been extremely proud of all her grandchildren, especially since she never finished school.

Society doesn't teach us how to grieve, and those who have yet to experience it think that grief is a linear process. But I have seen how the stages of grief can collapse into a jumble, how grief has no time line, and how important it is to have minimal expectations about how we'll respond to grief when it inevitably arrives at our own door.

But we can hope to read the situation with agility, respond to others with empathy and find the courage to let go, thereby giving us a chance to emerge as whole.

In travelling through grief, the poet Rumi says it best: that we carry inside us the wonders we seek outside us.

Dr Ranjana Srivastava

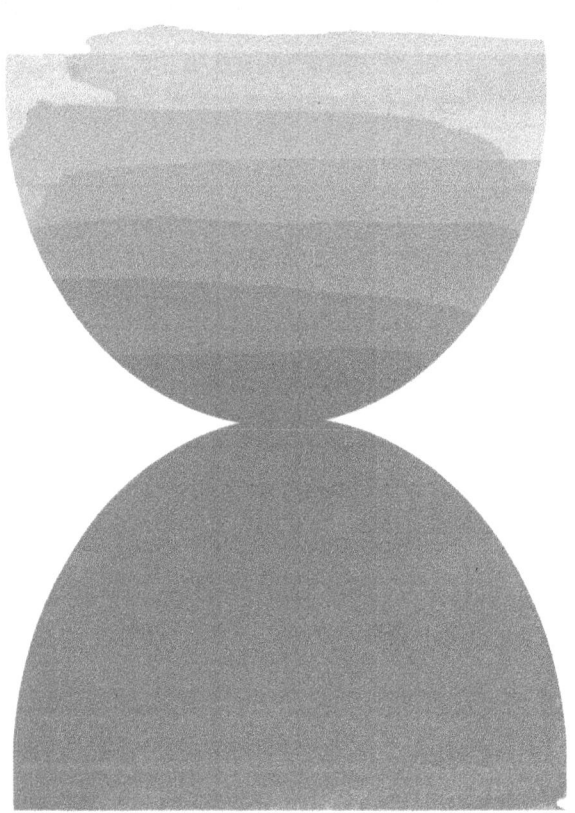

Friendship and grief

*If you have one true friend,
you have more than your share.*

Thomas Fuller

OVER THE PAST SIX YEARS, Josie had become a familiar face in the waiting room. After many ups and downs, her health was now failing. After being diagnosed with brain metastases, I knew that she was close to calling it an end to treatment and my heart felt heavy as I greeted her.

For the first time, she sat in a wheelchair, smiling but looking thin and tired. Josie was always grateful for something, even if it were the sun on a wintry morning or being seen in clinic without delay.

I suddenly realised that all these years Josie had been accompanied by the same woman who would see her to my door but never come inside.

'Who is that?' I asked curiously that day.

'Oh, that's Rae, my best friend.'

I'd heard many heartwarming stories of friendship but there was always room for more. While filling out a lengthy insurance form, I asked Josie to tell me about Rae.

She told me they'd met on the first day of school for their respective firstborns. After the children had gone inside, the two tearful mothers decided to take a walk.

They never looked back. Their children turned eighteen, twenty-one and then thirty and the two friends remained close.

At this, I recalled my own experience of meeting new parents at my children's primary school. Many of our conversations were short and the relationships felt transactional. We met over athletics and barbecues, but it took a leap of imagination to think that the adult friendships would outlast the time our children spent together. I marvelled to Josie that a friendship that started at the school gates and thrived decades later was a testament to their character. She beamed at the compliment.

Josie had lost her husband a few years earlier and was left with two daughters who lived nearby and were increasingly responsible for managing Josie's home affairs while Rae saw to the medical aspects. Hearing this, I encouraged Josie to bring Rae into the appointments with her.

A good friend is priceless but never more so than during a time of need – I liked Rae from the description but as I got to know her found even more to be impressed by.

As Josie's memory faltered, she relied on Rae to remember her questions and relay her daughters' concerns, but Rae had the rare knack of never making herself sound more important or more reliable than her friend. When Josie developed word-finding difficulties, Rae never interrupted or finished off her sentence, instead enabling her to continue. When Josie felt well, Rae prompted her to walk but when she looked tired, she insisted on using a wheelchair. On the day Josie finally decided that she no longer wanted to come back to clinic, Rae helped temper the finality of the decision by suggesting they spend more time at the beach, which cheered Josie. On that last visit, I wished Josie luck and told her I'd miss her. I also expressed my admiration for Rae, who replied simply, 'She'd have done the same for me.'

Rae stood by Josie in her final days and brought calm through her presence and ability to anticipate her needs. She also proved a pillar of support for her daughters, who grew in confidence as a result.

Watching deep friendships work naturally is a privilege, but it's more common for me to meet casual acquaintances and good friends who want to be helpful and don't know how. They fear saying something inappropriate or doing something wrong at a sensitive time and hesitate to offer suggestions that may be misconstrued.

Meanwhile, most patients would be grateful for help but hate to be a burden – we intrinsically value our dignity and independence.

It was my good friend Joy who showed me how to help someone who is not a close friend or relative.

When Joy's colleague, Eve, was suddenly diagnosed with a catastrophic illness and her co-workers were wondering how to help, Joy offered to take Eve's children home after school, take care of their dinner and supervise their homework before dropping them home. Inundated by appointments, Eve and her husband welcomed this relief and Joy became an anchor for their family. This arrangement lasted for several months until Eve became more unwell.

After discussions with her family, Joy extended her help to having Eve's children spend a few nights at her house during the most tumultuous phase of their life when their mother had to endure repeated hospital visits. I was sure that Joy's house was an oasis for the children but I was nevertheless curious to know how her husband and children reacted.

She told me that they'd agreed they had the resources and goodwill to help others and that, if the situation ever grew untenable, they'd review it. But given their resilience and generosity, it never did. Joy told me that they periodically asked about Eve but never probed the children, choosing to confine themselves to providing the normality they needed. I was struck by her emotional maturity.

Eve's condition continued to decline and within a year of diagnosis she was dying. I continued to learn from Joy's response to the situation. She admitted that, being non-medical, she didn't really understand the nuances of Eve's illness but also didn't need to know more than she was told. This proved prophetic because Eve was said to be bitter about her fate and unable to accept her deterioration. As a result, she had distanced herself from others, including her helpers.

I couldn't help admiring that, in spite of the fact that Joy received hardly any explicit recognition for her generosity, she took her role seriously, never judged, and focused on the children's welfare. She also had a full-time job and didn't overextend herself.

It was a fine balancing act and she acquitted it marvellously. As she explained it, she was playing a modest role in a great tragedy and just wanted to do her best. All of society is enriched by people like her.

At some point, we will all find our lives intermingled with those of our friends and acquaintances who are experiencing illness. Whereas some will count their blessings, many will lament the gradual erosion of friendship through unwanted advice, unwelcome intrusion and fixed ideas. Most people actually want to be a good friend to someone who is ill or dying but have never been taught how.

Here are some suggestions that everyone appreciates.

Be there in the ways they need

Death can happen within days or weeks or be slow and inexorable. For the patient, this phase of life may be a time of internal reflection, colliding thoughts and involuntary worries. For friends, a rapid death can be shocking, while a slow death unearths many questions and internal conflicts.

We may not know all the ways to comfort the dying or ourselves but simply being present is the most important act of kindness. The consolation of a hundred distracted text messages and group emails pales into insignificance before someone who shows up to say 'I am sorry about your news, I am here.'

We commonly worry about imposing on people we don't know well but most of us die feeling lonely rather than crowded by well-wishers. Someone grappling with difficult physical and emotional concerns doesn't lose the desire for human communion, but fulfilling this desire becomes difficult on one's own. My sickest patients constantly worry about not being able to reciprocate friendship and kindness. Something they really appreciate is replacing the open-ended offer 'Let me know if you need anything' with a more committed 'I'd like to see you but will stay only as long as you want.'

Dr Ranjana Srivastava

I tried this recently with a friend who is terminally ill. I brought lunch and was confident of not overstaying my welcome. But I'd forgotten how easily she tired and was mortified when she had to tell me to go. Embarrassed by my lack of sensitivity, I chastised myself for assuming that she'd wanted me there at all. But she sent me an email that very evening saying how much she had enjoyed seeing me and asking if I'd come again. I saw that, despite her reduced energy, she was still invested in our friendship.

Terminally ill patients are often bombarded by questions from professionals, caregivers and complete strangers. Good friends avoid this, instead finding ways of simply being present.

When a widower was struggling to look after himself at home, I asked why he didn't tell his many concerned neighbours how to help. He sighed that he had to find something that sounded important, although his greatest wish was for someone to warm his food and read the newspaper to him.

Another very valuable support is a concrete offer to complete some household chores that don't stop for anyone. No help is too menial and just being there fosters understanding.

Be willing to listen

A ninety-year-old patient once gave me some unforgettable advice. He said that all he wanted at the end of life was for someone to listen. He didn't want his condition to be compared with others and didn't need stories of survival. He didn't need to hear he was courageous or that he would be fine. He wasn't afraid to die but, while alive, all he yearned for was companionship that was quiet and undemanding and capable of handling the inevitable sadness of getting old and feeble. When faced with the question of how to help a dying friend, this is advice we can all use.

Build a team

Supporting someone at the end of life is hard, even for the trained. It's not meant to be a solitary task, no matter how much determination and capability we bring to it. Wherever possible, we should enable others to join us in the journey.

Being mindful of one's own commitments isn't selfish, rather it's sensible, and we can care for each other more efficiently if we build a team with assigned tasks. However, it's crucial to be considerate of the patient's actual needs. For instance, many of my patients are plied with food at a time when their appetite is poor and their freezer crammed with uneaten meals. They feel ungrateful declining more meals but, if someone asked them, they'd love for their pet to be walked, their bed to be made, or to go on a drive.

We should want the dying to trust that we are not out to change their whole lives and that no job is too small for us.

Being a friend who aims to fulfil these needs is our chance to care meaningfully for the dying.

Recognise it won't always be easy

The impending loss of a friend is heartbreaking but the act of caring for someone at the end of life is also one of the most fulfilling acts we are called upon to do in life. While we all aspire to a peaceful end, it's common for everyone involved to suffer crises of confidence. Hope, despondency, relief and anxiety can all cycle together – good friends understand this and rise to the challenge. They know when to advocate and when to be silent. Friends must find ways of pacing themselves, acknowledge their own fears and frustrations, and locate their own supports.

There is no need to downplay the challenge of our work or the emptiness the death of a friend will generate; we could embrace our role knowing that we are made stronger by caring for others and take heart in the consolations of a friendship we have honoured to the end.

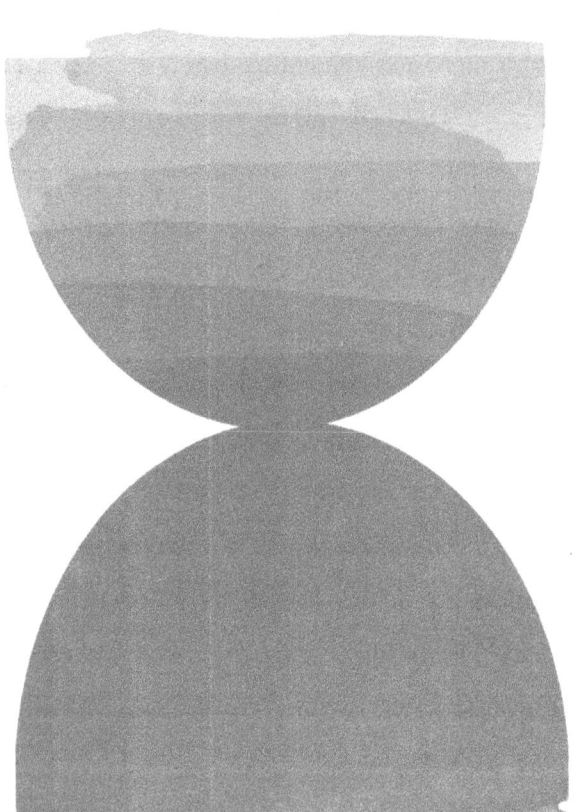

Deciding between work and rest

Sometimes the most important thing in a whole day is the rest we take between two deep breaths.

Etty Hillesum

MANY PATIENTS DIAGNOSED with a serious illness face a dilemma. They aren't entirely well, but their prognosis isn't immediately poor, and statistics can't predict how an individual patient will fare.

Being sick is costly and stressful. Healthcare expenses build up, the mortgage still needs to be paid, the bills keep coming and the family still needs to eat. For many people it's necessary to keep working, but beyond income, work serves another purpose. At a time when our identity is challenged on a number of fronts, work can be an anchor. Colleagues can become friends and willing supporters. A project and a deadline can be a welcome distraction from the anxieties of life. Talking to people battling their own problems can help us realise that we are not alone in our predicament.

Upon receiving a diagnosis of advanced cancer, the first thing Yasmin did was to resign from her office job. Overwhelmed by events, she submitted her resignation on the way to her first chemotherapy appointment, saying she couldn't think of ever wanting to return to work.

I was sympathetic but wished she had waited a little or used her ample sick leave. As it turned out, she responded to treatment and her symptoms improved – and while she needed prolonged treatment, she wasn't dying as soon as she had feared. This left Yasmin with a lot of free time. With a husband working full-time and her children grown, Yasmin began experiencing something she hadn't imagined: boredom. This led to hours spent on internet chat groups, which fuelled severe anxiety.

Yasmin was a medical receptionist who'd enjoyed her work. She reflected that contact with patients would have helped her maintain perspective as she experienced her own illness, and I agreed, but she'd been replaced, and it was next to impossible to find a new job in her situation.

Her illness was classified as terminal because it was incurable but she was experiencing the next best alternative, long-term control. Thanks to modern medicine, there are many people like Yasmin with previously untreatable diseases who are living longer and better lives. They do live under a cloud of uncertainty and their life expectancy is shortened compared to a healthy population, but they're grateful that their illness is not the immediate death sentence it used to be.

The social worker helped Yasmin find an exercise group for cancer patients, which inspired her to become a qualified trainer for the organisation. Yasmin had seven good years following her diagnosis, much of it made possible by finding a purpose.

When the initial panic of discovering an incurable illness has abated, I often find myself having conversations with my patients about work.

A few people come to mind then, including my friend Bob, a teacher who worked with disadvantaged youth. The students assigned to him came from broken homes and backgrounds of substance abuse, intergenerational poverty and, sometimes, plain bad luck. Bob had to devise a solution to encourage each child to stay in school. He told me that sometimes it simply meant buying the child a new pair of shoes, so he wouldn't be teased, or playing a game of basketball to diffuse anger. I was chastened by his comment that securing a child's safety was more important than getting homework done.

Bob's diabetes slowly resulted in end-stage renal failure just before he turned eighty, at which point he elected not to undergo dialysis. Given months to live, he replied that this was enough time to hand over his duties to other volunteers.

I'd always found Bob's work challenging, but was moved by his willingness to keep working with his students even as he dealt with his own mortality. For him, dying didn't mean giving up on life and he needed purpose to the end. His fitness had diminished but he knew that even small things like listening attentively, reducing conflict and teaching perseverance mattered. Helping children was his way of expressing gratitude for his life.

I'd worried that the stresses of his work would diminish Bob's capacity to cope with his own situation but I saw that helping others was Bob's form of self-care. On days he felt flat or unmotivated, he only had to go to work to put his problem in perspective. Sometimes, being busy at work can be an excuse to avoid dealing with important matters, but not so for Bob. He worked for four months before relinquishing his badge at a fond farewell. His daughter moved in and he died peacefully at home, as he'd wanted.

Yasmin and Bob were people who wanted to work and derived meaning from it. But many people diagnosed with a terminal illness are retired, unable or unfit to work. Among my younger, seriously ill patients have been an interstate truck-driver who didn't have the stamina to work, a principal who could not switch to flexible hours, a machine operator who couldn't take morphine and work safely and a chief executive who couldn't afford to take extended sick leave. Other patients believe that they have more important priorities than working and it's not hard to see why.

Finally, there are people who need more rest but find themselves left with no quality of life while on a treadmill of medical interventions. A dialysis patient was exhausted by spending every day in some part of the hospital. Another young patient had severe heart failure and was tired of expecting a reversal of fortune at every hospitalisation. Amid the focus on their disease, the conversation that was missing was one about accepting mortality and defining how they wanted to live the remainder of their life. Once these patients met the palliative care team, they changed their outlook, wound down futile medical procedures, and eventually died at home.

There is no single answer to balancing work and rest when one is diagnosed with a terminal illness – it depends on many considerations, chiefly how well someone feels. Troubling physical symptoms such as pain or fatigue make it logistically difficult to work. On the other hand, people who feel physically well and emotionally robust might choose to work, especially in a flexible environment. Occasionally, when clearly unwell patients insist on working till the very end of life, they can inconvenience their colleagues and impact their loved ones, who are denied an opportunity for closure. This is something that calls for self-awareness.

Our work is important but it cannot disguise the existential questions that are at the heart of dying well. We must find our own meaning via contemplation and through communion with those who care about us. I have yet to meet a dying patient who grieves not working harder or keeping longer hours, but countless people have regretted compromised friendships, broken relationships and losing their bearings. We all have something to learn from those who don't let their work define them.

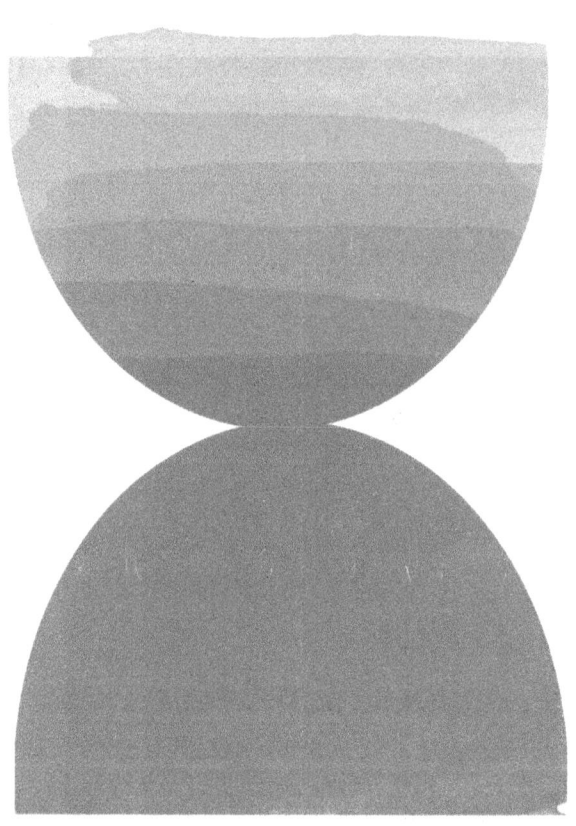

Caring for a loved one with dementia

From caring comes courage.
Lao Tzu

MY FRIEND KIM AND I attended medical school together and later trained together, too. Every week during medical school we travelled long distances to reach our assigned hospitals. Such close proximity either bares differences or brings us closer. We remain good friends, although these days our children's lives take precedence over anatomy specimens.

I jokingly attribute my loyalty to Kim to her mother's generosity towards me. My parents lived abroad and I had to be self-sufficient from an early age. I managed a busy university schedule, laundry, rent and bills. I had a part-time job, and never exceeded my budget, but the hardest thing was cooking for one person. I had a well-stocked library but an empty pantry.

Kim lived at home and was looked after in the same way my parents would have looked after me. Her mother was a nurse – practical, capable, and no-nonsense. When we first met, she didn't ask me what I ate or how I managed. Noting her daughter's busy student life, she put the rest together. This led to her pressing a bag of food containers into my hands on many occasions when I visited. I felt self-conscious, but she had such a natural manner that the gesture felt easy and I was always grateful.

As if this weren't enough, on my overlapping night shifts with Kim she'd pack me dinner.

Night shifts usually evoke images of squandered sleep and emergency dashes, but one of my enduring memories is that of Kim and I finding respite from a hectic night of work and sampling her mother's cooking under a bright moon. Such was the measure of a woman who received nothing but silent thanks in return.

Kim and I graduated, got older, and passed other milestones. I visited less frequently but always came away with a token of her mother's cooking, including tubs of soup to restore me after childbirth. She never stopped being thoughtful, which is why it came as such a shock when I first heard the news that her mind might be failing her.

Shortly afterwards, I met her mother at a wedding. Her unblemished face and slender build were recognisable, but her eyes seemed distant when she smiled at me. I watched her husband guide her protectively towards the bathroom. I'd met so many patients like her but before then I'd never imagined that someone I knew would be rapidly afflicted by dementia.

On my occasional visits to their house, Kim's father now took the lead role of greeting me and inviting me in. She was often asleep or resting quietly in a chair, a far cry from the bustling woman of my student days who was never far from the stovetop. She'd still ask after my children but couldn't remember their birth order, which sounded hardly surprising considering she didn't see them often.

And then one day, she didn't know who I was. Neither examining my face nor her husband's subtle hints prompted her memory. I felt sad then, but it was her eventual failure to ply me with food that marked the end of an era.

After the diagnosis of dementia, Kim and her father ably looked after her mother for many years. I was privileged to watch closely how Kim dealt with the challenge of a parent facing the onslaught of progressive dementia.

Kim made it a point to visit her mother regularly even though meaningful interaction became scarce. Every week without fail, Kim drove her parents to a familiar lunch spot, recognising the consolations of a familiar ritual. The conversation didn't flow as freely but I knew how much they looked forward to the date because Kim's father always mentioned it when I saw him. Kim's mother had always been proud of the doctor in the family but what really lit up her life was the presence of her daughter.

The family had expected to care for her at home but as often happens, the reality didn't match expectations and Kim's mother needed residential care. By this time, she was experiencing mood disturbances where her apparent placidity would suddenly change to uncharacteristic aggression. There were remonstrations, accusations and pleas with inexplicable content and context. Dementia chipped away relentlessly at her personality, wringing out the patience, sweetness and goodwill that she was loved for. The dramatic changes were confronting, but Kim's allegiance never wavered and she continued to show up every week to see her mother. Many of those times it must have felt as if her mother had been replaced by a stranger, but Kim strived to make the best of the situation and never turned away.

As doctors, we had both seen families embarrassed or distressed by the unpredictable behaviour of dementia sufferers and understood why some relatives couldn't bear to visit. What I most admired about Kim was her unspoken determination to separate the person from the disease and keep up her visits through mounting heartache.

Then suddenly, as if this tragedy wasn't enough, Kim's mother lost her capacity to speak. In one of the most devastating turns of fate, she would stay alive for many years without being able to communicate. She grew passive and more pliant. Sometimes, such obvious slowing hastens demise but not this time. Kim's mother lived in this unrecognisable state for years, so with a knot in my stomach, I watched in awe as Kim navigated the most grievous of circumstances. Two things stayed in my mind from the experience.

When an ailing parent enters residential care, there is an unspoken expectation that family members will take turns to provide additional care and presence beyond that of paid carers. While we might expect facilities to cater for all our loved ones' needs, the reality is that this doesn't happen. Even when basic requirements such as food, hygiene and safety are well met, most residents spend their days and nights alone.

Kim understood the limitations of her mother's facility and also knew that her mother was among the most vulnerable of patients, unable to participate in any communal activities or be entertained by volunteers. In fact, there was little anyone could do except sit quietly and be a familiar presence. In an era when we panic at the thought of momentary quiet, sitting for hours with a parent who has lost the capacity for self-expression must be one of the hardest things to bear, yet Kim did it unquestioningly. I marvelled that this was never out of obligation but an innate confidence that it was how she wished to remember her final acts towards her mother.

Sometimes, I'd tell Kim about warring families I met at work whom I wondered how to help. She told me that she had just one creed: to care for her mother to the best of her capacity and focus on her own actions. I saw this when she brought in small gifts such as a single flower and took her young children to visit their grandmother every week. She wanted them to have a memory of her even though it wasn't clear if she recognised them.

I always thought this to be Kim's finest achievement – her ability to do what was right without worrying about what others thought actually won her the freedom from the disagreements that can rock families. As Oscar Wilde said, 'To give and not expect return, that is what lies at the heart of love.'

Kim's father spent every day at his wife's bedside and dedicated himself to her care. Still youthful and interested in the world, this was an enormous undertaking but one he performed with grace and devotion. But he also longed for the spouse he no longer had. Kim's second, and to my mind even trickier balancing act, was to not judge her father for wanting another companion. Not only this, she also stood by him as he entered another relationship. She must have felt conflicted, but again, she had a mature grasp of essential human needs. His choices were not her battle to fight. Instead, she focused on what she could influence, a kind and understanding relationship with her father.

Dr Ranjana Srivastava

Kim's mother died quietly some years ago. Her funeral was small and private, a remembrance of her vitality and relief at her passing. For me, her death meant a further pulling away from a part of my youth that had been illuminated by her generosity.

Some years have passed since her death and what strikes me is Kim's equanimity, which I attribute to her conduct during the troubled times. Kim always says that she wasn't heroic or extraordinary; instead, she reconciled herself to the truth of her mother's illness, defined what she could control, and fulfilled her duties. Accepting that there was more than one way of seeing a situation allowed her to avoid conflict and stay calm and poised.

Kim was no more born with these traits than the rest of us, but her mother's dementia forced her to contend with new ideas. Kim was determined to live wisely and be a role model to her children. She got there by being true to herself and, in the process, taught me an unforgettable lesson in how to behave honourably towards the dying.

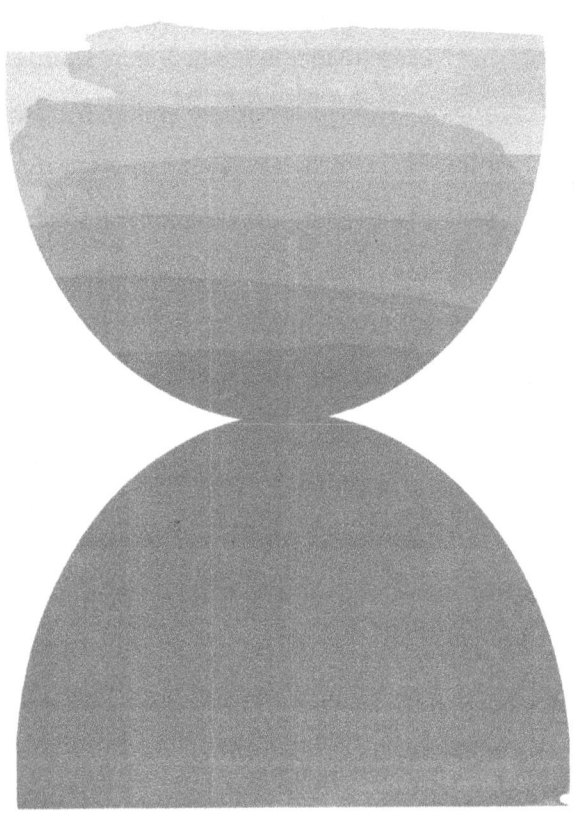

Helping our loved ones die comfortably

*Ever has it been that love knows not its own depth
until the hour of separation.*

Khalil Gibran

THERE WAS A COMPLAINT BREWING and the nurse wanted me to nip it in the bud, so on a weekend morning I found myself sitting down with Tara, the granddaughter of an elderly man brought from a nursing home with pneumonia.

Tara looked about thirty. Her grandfather was one hundred years old. It happens once or twice a year but meeting a centenarian never fails to trigger my awe as I wonder about all the things packed into that lifetime.

Tara looked tired, with rings around her eyes. Her crumpled clothes suggested she'd spent the night sitting up with her grandfather. This was no easy undertaking for anyone and

I was touched by her consideration. Her grandfather looked semi-conscious. His breaths came slowly but his expression was peaceful, and he looked comfortably propped up on two pillows.

But Tara declared that the night nurse had been 'terrible' and not administered enough morphine. I was disheartened because no relative should have to worry about inadequate care at the end of life.

'We certainly don't want him in pain,' I reassured her. 'Is he comfortable right now?'

'Yes, but I'm worried about tonight if he has the same nurse.'

Pain relief should be taken seriously, whether after a fall, a fracture, or at the end of life.

I was puzzled since I knew the nurse to be experienced and thought she would have been my pick to care for a dying patient. Reassuring Tara that I'd handle the matter, I was wondering what to do next when the nurse found me. She didn't know about the complaint but appeared upset and asked me for advice about an overnight encounter.

She related the story of an unconscious elderly man whose granddaughter wanted him to have more morphine when other charted medications had been more appropriate. However, the granddaughter had accused her of being uncaring, which had shaken her.

'Why do you think Tara was upset?' I gently enquired.

'She wanted things over quickly. I know how she felt because I sat with my mother recently and thought her death would never come. But I'd never deprive someone of pain relief.'

When I checked the charts, I saw that the patient had received morphine and other drugs at appropriate intervals, and by other reports, too, had remained comfortable. He died later that day and I called Tara afterwards to express my condolences and arrange a meeting to discuss her complaint, but she was no longer interested.

'The nurse was probably right. I was tired and I don't want to think about it anymore.'

Tara may have moved on but I saw the toll the complaint took on the nurse, whose confidence was shaken for months afterwards. A claim of negligence at the end of life is a serious personal and professional matter, but the real problem wasn't the lack of morphine. It was the fact that Tara had never seen anyone close to her die and didn't know how to react. This is an increasingly common problem encountered by professionals.

The very next week, however, there was a genuinely troubling complaint from two siblings who had been at the bedside of their terminally ill father for two days. Their father's consciousness had deteriorated but the intended morphine infusion was never started due to a lack of communication and poor follow-up over a holiday weekend.

I began with an apology for their experience and assured them that appropriate palliation shouldn't have to wait. The infusion was started, an intern and a junior nurse were reminded of their duty to escalate matters beyond their expertise and the siblings were satisfied. In fact, they emphasised their motivation to help other patients avoid a similar ordeal. We were all impressed by their grace and forbearance.

These two accounts showed me that terminal care can suffer due to reasons of expectation, understanding and communication. We can be firm advocates for the dying but also accept that we may not always be right. The death of a loved one is one of life's most stressful occasions and bereavement triggers complex emotions. Managing our own emotions and accepting the reality of death is often the key to allowing others to die well.

Tara's grandfather was actually receiving good end-of-life care, but she needed a better explanation of the dying process. The siblings were right to demand better care and not accept the status quo. It can be difficult for loved ones to speak up and healthcare systems must be better equipped to anticipate barriers to good end-of-life care.

Dr Ranjana Srivastava

FAMILIARISING OURSELVES with palliative care services early in the course of a terminal illness is one way to help ourselves and our loved ones die comfortably. Palliative care does not hasten death; it troubleshoots symptoms and elevates emotional well-being. It improves the quality of remaining life and the experience of dying and in some cases, meticulous palliative care even prolongs life. Research shows that experiencing a good death reduces the immediate anxiety and stress of family members and influences their view of their own mortality.

Obstacles to palliative care include a lack of access but also a perception that it means giving up. Where palliative care is regarded as a last-ditch measure, people come to it too late. But when we accept the notion that we are mortal and permit ourselves to focus on what matters, palliative care can make a difference. I'd be the first to say that palliative care cannot fulfil every expectation of every patient but if we want to die well, we must begin from a place of honesty and reflection and believe that dying well is as important as living well.

I commonly meet adults in their thirties and forties who have never seen someone close to them die and are overwhelmed by their first encounter of death. The collision of sadness, guilt and helplessness are all too human but if we have never thought about being mortal, we will fail to prioritise the needs of the dying.

As a student watching deaths made worse by disagreements amongst relatives, I often used to wonder why doctors just didn't take charge. With time, I have realised that this is virtually impossible without the instructions of the patient or the consent of relatives.

Such is the momentum of medicine to intervene that even slight hesitation has the power to stall end-of-life care. Common examples include withdrawing antibiotics, withholding chest compressions, and stopping artificial nutrition.

I can recall many instances where actions guided by emotion not fact have led to decisions that have not prolonged survival but prevented a peaceful death. Increasingly, dying well requires a concerted effort for all parties to unite. We owe this to the people who rely on us.

The role of assisted dying

Euthanasia, or voluntary assisted dying, is often in the news these days and this is an appropriate place to talk about it because, for some people, a good death may need to be an assisted one.

Assisted dying is legal in various international jurisdictions and the law will come into effect in the Australian state of Victoria in June 2019.

The specific eligibility criteria that patients must meet to request access to assisted dying are important but broadly speaking, a patient must be deemed by several experts to be suffering from an incurable, advanced and progressive disease that will lead to an imminent and inevitable death. To request assisted dying in Victoria, patients must be over the age of 18 and have decision-making capacity. Mental illness and disability alone are not grounds for a request and patients must satisfy all other criteria. There is no provision for people to leave instructions about assisted dying in an advance care directive, and no one else can initiate a request on the patient's behalf.

Once approved, the patient is prescribed medication that causes sedation, paralysis and death. The process is usually quick and painless. In some places, the patient must swallow the medication; in others, a helper is permitted to administer oral medication, or a doctor can inject a lethal drug. The death can happen at home or, in some instances, a facility.

Wherever assisted dying has been mooted, it has not been without furious debate. To its advocates, it means an end to the suffering associated with death and dying. It honours an individual's dignity and avoids prolonging the inevitable. The evidence thus far shows that most patients who are prescribed the medication don't use it but value the security of having an option to end their life if their suffering becomes unbearable.

To its detractors, assisted dying presents moral and practical challenges. Is it ever right to deliberately end a life?

Who decides that a life is not worth living? Can patients who feel like a burden be coerced to die? How can doctors loyally save lives and end lives?

At its heart, assisted dying questions the meaning we attach to our lives and what we consider to be a life worth living.

As someone whose professional life revolves around the subject of dying, I am deeply interested in helping people achieve a better, less fearful death and accept that assisted dying may be a part of this. However, I make the following observations.

The vast majority of my patients are afraid of the symptoms associated with dying, particularly pain but also nausea, confusion and fatigue. They mourn the loss of independence and with it, dignity. Many ward off the thought of dying and fear to discuss it openly. Their worst imaginings added to the myths they hear push them into a spiral of anxiety. Above all else, such people require comfort and reassurance. Palliative care does not eradicate every symptom, rarely banishes all existential distress and, in some people, simply falls short of its goals, but it helps more people in more ways to have a better death.

In all my years of being an oncologist, people have pleaded with me every day to prolong life but have rarely asked to end life. For those rare patients, life had truly become not worth living, but what's compelling to me is that so many others, faced with declining health and an existence that observers may find unacceptable, express an affinity for life and its myriad offerings.

Growing older has helped me understand that people who are well are not always well-suited to judge the lives of the seriously ill. For some of my sickest patients, whose lives might be dismissed as empty, simply sitting in their garden watching people go by or receiving a visit from a grandchild is a profound source of contentment. My youngest patients hadn't bargained for premature death but, in the throes of a terminal illness, still hang on to a family's embrace and the aroma of a home-cooked meal. Some patients demand full cognitive and physical capacity as a precondition to a good life; many adjust to more modest expectations.

Utterly humbled by my learning, I no longer assume and always ask, 'What does life mean to you?'

Assisted dying is always going to be a deeply personal and philosophical exercise. Doctors should strive to serve the patient's best interest and ensure that people are equipped to make important decisions about how to die. This includes providing clear and non-judgmental information about assisted dying.

Our choices will vary but even before we arrive there, we must think carefully, choose wisely and not be afraid to believe that we can achieve a better death.

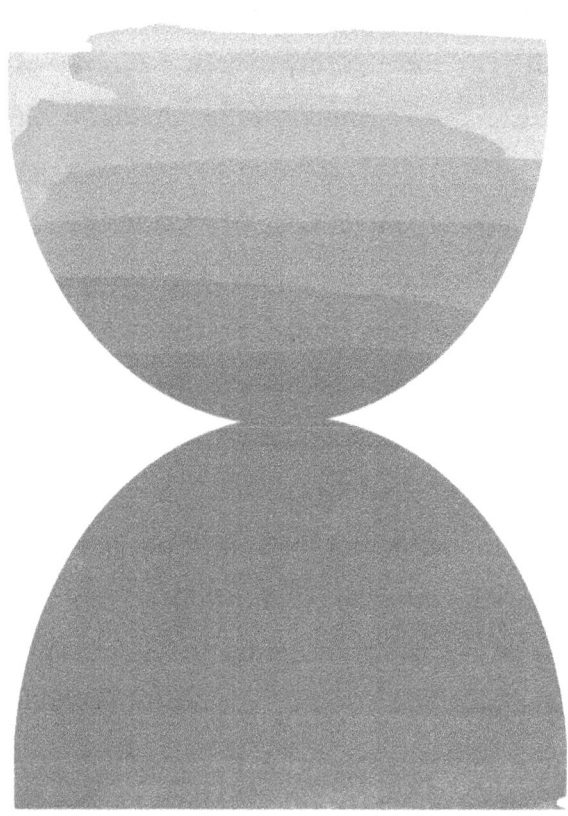

Being a good advocate for the dying

In the end we only regret the chances we didn't take.
Anonymous

I RECENTLY ATTENDED A TALK in which a veteran intensive care physician declared that in nearly fifty years of patient care, he had yet to encounter a good death. With the audience suitably startled, he proceeded to explain that judicious decisions could often avoid futile care and allow the patient to die peacefully but even then, the reality of human lives is such that there is always someone left behind. Truly, if we consider all the people involved in our lives who might be impacted by our death, the notion of a good death doesn't seem as clean-cut. In particular, the doctor reflected, he felt sympathetic towards the staunchest advocates who felt the loss most keenly.

Listening to him, I thought of my own patients. When they died, their loved ones knew at an intellectual level that their suffering had come to an end, but it didn't stop them from mourning the loss and wishing it weren't so. If their relationship had been rich and generous, they simply longed for the deceased; if the bonds were frayed, they regretted not having the chance to do better.

Sometimes, in a twist of fate, I end up caring for the terminally ill spouse or a close relative of a deceased patient. I am conscious that seeing me again must bring back sad memories, but I am touched to hear patients say that they are consoled by a familiar face. This has allowed me to observe that how people cope with their own decline is intimately associated with how they helped a loved one navigate the end of life.

As the bereaved know, there is no protocol for navigating loss, but there are some things it helps to remember.

We should keep the focus on the dying person, something obvious to say but easy to overlook. There's a time to set aside differences and aim for quiet reflection, calm and – where necessary – open forgiveness. It may be too late to expect long discussions and significant decisions.

One of the hardest things I found was deciding how much of my life to share with a dear friend who was slowly dying. As she grew progressively weaker, I was still involved in interesting activities that she loved but could no longer do.

After vacillating between feeling insensitive at revealing too much and disingenuous for withholding things, I cautiously started sharing my experiences and was pleasantly surprised to find how much she enjoyed a normal conversation that treated her like a person.

I have also learnt that, as important as it is to be agile in conversation, it's vital to know when to be quiet. The latter is something most of us find hard, but people at the end of life often lack the energy to be an attentive host. Nevertheless, they are consoled by company and satisfied by feeling included in the human chain even if they don't say much.

We know a lot about welcoming a newborn to the world but struggle to tend the dying.

I sometimes field calls from people who are anxious about visiting someone at the end of life. Close friends and family members suddenly feel tongue-tied and even professionals can feel tense. But we should know that it's possible to overcome our hesitation and create meaningful exchange.

The art of any conversation lies in recognising cues. We are not obliged to be falsely jovial or unnecessarily distracting and, in fact, it's perfectly reasonable to ask how we can make ourselves useful. For instance, we might be better at reading aloud and telling jokes or we'd prefer to file bills and prune the roses. The key is being present and being attentive. These are valuable tips for nurturing any relationship but especially those at the end of life where there is an imbalance of power between the patient and the caregiver.

I once looked after a terminally ill widow who was acutely aware of her nephews' apprehensions at every visit. To encourage them to keep coming, she assigned small tasks to each one such as opening her mail, folding her laundry, and massaging her feet. She laughed that the jobs helped dissipate their nervousness and made their visits enjoyable. The nephews were proud of their contribution and I admired her alacrity in shaping her circumstances.

A young woman I knew had always been the life of social events but when she had a serious accident with life-threatening complications, her friends banded together to hold small parties at her house. She joined them when she felt well, otherwise would happily rest in a chair. She regularly hailed the joy she found in her friends' gesture and I thought that her friends would always be proud of creating a meaningful ritual to sustain them through difficult times.

Families should be mindful that even experts can feel strained when looking after the dying. I once knew a young woman, Kara, whose parents were determined to take her home. On the night Kara died, the community nurse assigned to attend her happened to be on one of her first independent shifts and became visibly upset at the sight. The nurse called for help and made Kara comfortable, but not before her parents were distressed by the thought that they had deprived Kara of expert care by bringing her home. I explained to them that sometimes the professional detachment people expect can falter for very human reasons but Kara had benefited from the family's love and unity.

Appropriate, skilled and compassionate care at the end of life should be a basic right and we should strive to ensure that the dying receive the best possible care by advocating for those who cannot advocate for themselves.

We can speak quietly and purposefully about what our loved ones need. We must possess the facts and understand that being tired or stressed as a caregiver does not excuse hostility or violence towards professionals, which is becoming a noticeable problem in healthcare. Calculating the urgency of a request is always helpful. For instance, prompt pain-relief is critical, but a leaky shower can hardly be fixed overnight. Many people desire a private room but not everyone can get one and staff have a duty to prioritise.

When we think of advocating for the vulnerable and dying, we would do well to remember that the most meaningful gestures are not grand; often they are exceedingly humble.

Those who earn the gratitude of the dying tend to be those who apply balm to their dry lips, stroke their feet, adjust their pillows, bring their drink a little closer, and are willing to simply sit by the bedside. To care is to be present.

Another area where advocates can make a crucial difference is in helping dying patients avoid futile care. A colleague of mine once cared for a man who was estranged from his family and found himself struggling to make some serious decisions. His neighbour noted his predicament and offered to help. I heard how the neighbour's mere presence and her gentle probing helped elicit the patient's values and enabled him to make a confident decision to enter hospice.

No one likes to see a loved one struggle and many of us want to be an advocate but are afraid of not understanding the language of medicine. But this isn't what patients need. The best advocates listen to people. They use their acumen to ask thoughtful questions that shine the spotlight on the best interest of the patient. They object when necessary but realise that the best way to help is through dialogue.

Healthcare is full of people who know what to do. Advocates help us decide whether it's the right thing to do.

In order to avoid conflict at the end of life, it's important for each one of us to have thought ahead about what we want. At our most vulnerable and weak, we benefit from advocates who can contribute their knowledge, strength and temperament to our welfare. Therefore, we must appoint our advocates carefully and deliberately for there are few things more onerous than being asked to make highly consequential decisions that we didn't expect to make.

Dr Ranjana Srivastava

Advocating for our loved ones at the end of life is one of the most honourable tasks we can perform. With goodwill, foresight and a belief in the right of the dying to receive the best end-of-life care possible, we can look forward to acquitting ourselves with pride and satisfaction.

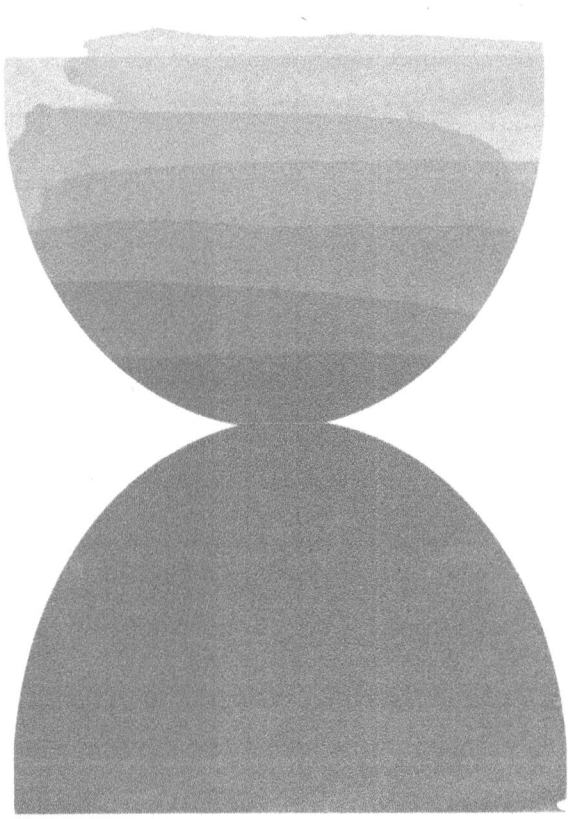

Ensuring the whole family gets help

A house divided cannot stand.
The New Testament

A FAMILY DOCTOR AND I were discussing the condition of a mutual patient who had resolutely declined community services including palliative care despite the inexorable progression of his disease.

'You know, he doesn't believe he is sick,' she said.

'He has an incurable illness!' I protested.

'That's not what he hears at his appointments.'

'Well, that's unbelievable,' I countered. 'I keep telling him things look bad.'

'I'm just letting you know what he thinks,' she said. 'As far as he's concerned, you're all wrong.'

'But that's so irritating.'

'Don't worry, we're all talking to him.'

But it wasn't working, I fretted.

I recalled her stricken call, when she had sent her 45-year-old patient, Andy, for tests. Having chastised herself for over-investigating, she was horrified to find that he had cancer.

I remembered the first time I met Andy. He'd come with his wife while her parents sat in the waiting room distracting the couple's children. His face was white with shock and she barely spoke.

I advised him that fortunately his cancer was operable, and I'd do everything in my power to keep him well. He looked at me pleadingly and my heart melted. A week ago, the couple had been planning nothing more taxing than a vacation – now, their lives had taken an unimaginable turn.

After his surgery, Andy received chemotherapy with great struggle. Consequently, he was overjoyed when, nearly a year since diagnosis, he was finished with treatment. Patients attend their first post-treatment visit with much anticipatory dread and while it's difficult to predict at that early visit who will go on to enjoy long-term good health, it's important to commend patients on their achievement. I did this and promised to keep a close eye on Andy, not knowing that his cancer would return just months later, exhibiting a vengeance that made me fear for his survival. I lacked the will and words to express the foreboding.

Dr Ranjana Srivastava

'The scans worry me,' I finally murmured.

'I know you'll fix it,' he said.

Andy's confidence never faltered, even when things started going wrong, and he defiantly assumed the challenge of outliving his prognosis. On one hand, his will was admirable; on the other hand, it was exhausting, especially for his relatives, who saw the deterioration he refused to admit.

Andy received every available treatment but within a few months his liver began failing, a radiologist glumly commenting that it contained more tumour than normal tissue.

I tried to talk to Andy about his future, but neither signal nor dialogue could dissuade him from believing that it was only a matter of time before I'd find a cure. Every doctor has a patient in denial who tests the boundaries, but this one was especially hard.

Inevitably, the day came when I thought it wasn't ethical to treat a patient in his weak state, but Andy put it down to a blip, because he was still able to run his business. Admittedly, an older patient would have felt much worse, but I feared that Andy was deceiving himself and not allowing his family to reconcile to his inevitable death.

Andy's wife, Mellie, was a psychologist who understood Andy's poor prognosis and his limited insight into the future. She wanted him to move towards acceptance, so they could prepare their family for a time without him. She was frustrated that, by avoiding any mention of dying, aggressively making future plans, and flatly rejecting palliative care input, he was stymying her efforts at preparing ahead.

Concerned, I turned to Andy's family doctor for help and witnessed a fine example of what a good relationship with the family doctor can achieve at the end of life.

Andy's doctor began by encouraging him in for a consultation instead of collecting scripts from the front desk, and she turned these occasions into a chance to explore Andy's understanding of his illness. Through attentive listening and sensitive probing, the doctor uncovered that his nonchalance concealed a mistrust of his specialists. He expressed a common fear among patients that missing even a single treatment due to fatigue would be seen as a sign of capitulation, which would prompt his doctors to give up on his care. As awkward as it was to hear what Andy thought, it helped me understand what I needed to do. The doctor and I began to speak regularly, underlining the one important thing that I couldn't offer Andy – a relationship that preceded his cancer diagnosis.

His doctor tactfully persuaded him to take a family holiday that he'd intended in the distant future. This turned out to be so enjoyable that it helped Andy concede he had an obligation to his family to help them cope with his illness. The ensuing relief opened his eyes to the silent grief that had been building around him and eventually opened the door to palliative care.

Dr Ranjana Srivastava

For the first time during his illness, he found a way to talk openly to his family, record memories for his children and wrap up his large business, which his wife had dreaded inheriting.

Like many young patients, Andy held on until late and then deteriorated rapidly, surprising everyone. I had often wondered how I'd go about managing his end-of-life care but the gentle perseverance of his family doctor and her rigorous emphasis on the whole family's welfare ensured that Andy accepted hospice and died there just days after admission. But thankfully, the family had come a long way by then.

The role of the hospital ended with Andy's death, but Mellie and her children benefited from community bereavement support and the ongoing involvement of a family doctor who'd accompanied them on an arduous journey. The doctor modestly said she'd played an ancillary role in tackling a great challenge but her involvement had been crucial in allowing Andy to experience a better death and smooth his family's path to recovery.

Apart from their daily work of preventing and treating illness, family doctors serve as a vital sounding board and I recommend that every patient find a good family doctor.

In an era of fast medicine, there's a noticeable divide. Many older patients have an established relationship with their doctor but younger people tend to go to rapid-service clinics lacking a fixed provider. A transactional relationship might work in the case of a common virus or a pulled muscle, but it lets us down when we face a deeper issue that demands time, engagement and a knowledge of the person behind the disease.

We're better served by not relying on hospitals to meet all our healthcare needs – this is why I urge patients to find a family doctor they can trust. Distance to the doctor's office and the language spoken by the doctor are important considerations at the end of life. As the first contact for community providers, the family doctor must also feel comfortable managing terminal illness.

Family doctors are committed to community-based care and want to help their patients die well. However, a lack of communication between specialists and family doctors can hamper this. A practical way to ensure that the family doctor is up to date is to request printed information at specialist visits and keep a file. In the case of unfolding diagnoses, sequential information can be extremely valuable.

A trusted relationship with a family doctor is desirable at any stage but it can transform our experience at the end of life. Confidence and control are ideas seldom associated with dying but we increase our chance of both by building a good relationship with our family doctor while we are well.

Dr Ranjana Srivastava

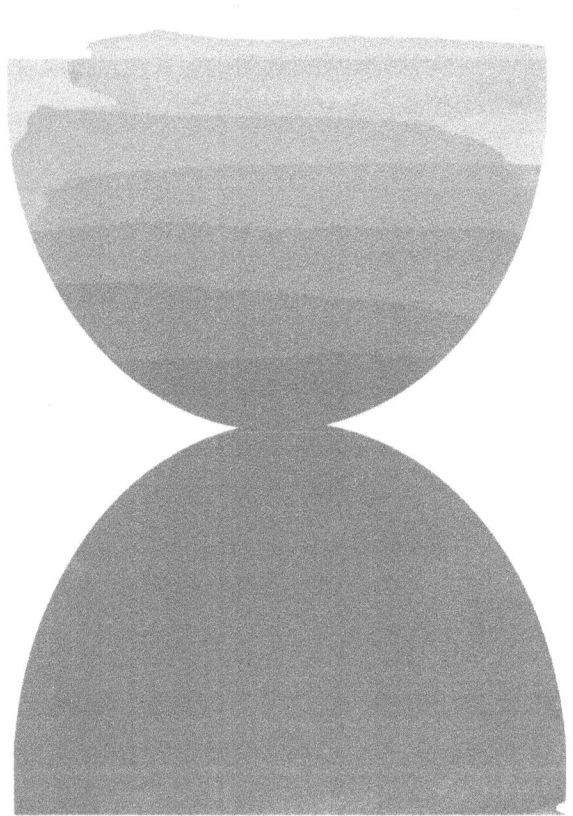

Planning ahead

*Live as if you were to die tomorrow;
learn as if you were to live forever.*

Mahatma Gandhi

'WHAT KIND OF A FUNERAL do you think she would have wanted?'

The question took me completely by surprise.

I don't know, I thought to myself. Should I know?

Victoria had been my patient for ten years. During this time, I had grown fond of her and could recount almost every detail of her journey. I could remember how I'd broken the news of disease progression, how she'd reacted, and how I'd studiously avoided agreeing with her on the miracles others kept mentioning. We weren't chasing miracles, I'd gently tell her, just good medicine and compassionate care.

Four months short of turning fifty, she was determined to celebrate her birthday in style although her body had been weakened by the ravages of disease. I told her honestly that having further chemotherapy would outweigh any benefit and, in the worst case, might even prevent her from reaching her milestone birthday. She replied that fifty was just half of where she intended to be.

Victoria turned fifty amid great fanfare and when I thumbed through the photos with genuine interest, I saw that it meant more to her than all the drugs I'd prescribed.

I was happy for her and thankful for her sister, Lisa, who had stepped down from a professional role to look after her. Lisa was curious, sensible and possessed of a calm that ably countered Victoria's anxiety.

At the end of every consultation, it's my habit to ask patients if there's anything else they wish to discuss – I often wished that Victoria would see fit to ask about her future, but all she ever requested was a copy of her results and an update on new therapies.

I was delighted when she once asked if she could fly abroad to visit an elderly aunt who had brought her up. Since I'd expressed increasing concern about her health, I thought perhaps she too was beginning to accept the situation. As I encouraged her to take a break from treatment and travel while she could, I hoped Lisa would throw in her support. Then I remembered that Lisa never intruded, as if she was determined to limit her role to supporting Victoria but not offering her opinion.

Victoria disliked making decisions; consequently, most things happened to her by default. However, as she neared the end of life, I wished her to make informed and deliberate decisions to help her live thoughtfully and die well. After debating the matter for three weeks, Victoria was unable to decide on travel and continued treatment. I fretted that I had fallen short of communicating her poor prognosis but all I could do was leave the door open for dialogue.

Sometime later, Victoria began losing her balance. She attributed it to her sleeping pills, but I gently revealed my suspicion of brain metastases. Indeed, an urgent scan confirmed my suspicion, but Victoria completely surprised me by saying she didn't want me to tell her the result at all. Usually, I support the right of patients to know as much or as little as they desire, but in this instance, I knew that a lack of disclosure would lead to uninformed decisions.

These issues present a real dilemma for doctors. With a patient's assent, family members can play an important role in easing fear and tackling avoidance. Lisa, however, showed no such inclination and while I acknowledged her regard for Victoria's autonomy, I regretted its consequence.

But it actually never struck me that a series of events, which included Victoria's visible decline, my decision to halt treatment, her idea to stop attending clinic, and the increased involvement of the palliative care team, would not add up to the fact for either sister that Victoria was terminally ill.

Then she died suddenly one night from a brain haemorrhage, and it was the morning after this that Lisa called me, asking my advice on Victoria's funeral.

'I just don't know what she'd have wanted,' she cried.

I was simply floored. Despite being so close, the sisters had never discussed this and, while it would have been a difficult conversation to have, Lisa's genuine bewilderment now was no less heart-wrenching.

I was dismayed to watch Lisa go about the task of arranging the funeral, having to contend with her own loss and the tricky logistics. Lisa felt alienated from Victoria's church, which she thought had aggressively distracted her from the idea of death. There was no private note or will, and Victoria's closest friends were not any wiser to her intimate wishes. I felt embarrassed that, despite countless visits, I was in the same boat.

Engulfed in sorrow and experiencing a touch of resentment, Lisa spent days arranging a funeral service befitting her sister. Taking her responsibility seriously, she trawled through archives, letters and personal effects to discover Victoria's core beliefs. I attended the funeral to pay my respects and was impressed by her effort but it was obvious to see the substantial emotional burden Lisa had to shoulder alone. From the stories of others, I imagined she would have a long journey to recovery.

To this day, I grapple with how complicated Victoria's death was despite the many years leading up to it, and what I could have done better. Unfortunately, her story matches those of many patients.

It's in our nature to avoid upsetting the people we love – and love commonly accompanies denial. But I have learnt that when we spend our entire lives without ever contemplating our mortality and giving our loved ones a window into our thoughts and desires, we risk leaving them a burdensome legacy.

The bereaved are left to wrestle with poignant questions. Did they miss saying something? Could they have done better? Did they do the deceased justice?

Victoria's death should be a cautionary tale for us all. Not even the most well-intentioned and caring professional can compel us to dwell on their mortality and most professionals would rather avoid the issue too. Therefore, ultimately, this is a task that falls to the individual.

To care about our loved ones means thinking about the toll that our death will exact on them and help them prepare as best as they can.

Some of my patients have movingly taken care of the smallest detail, such as clearing their wardrobe and donating their belongings, but at least, we owe it those left behind to mourn us without anxiety and second thoughts.

What would we want in the twilight of our life? What matters most? What might be our legacy? Such questions should empower us to lead our life deliberately. If not for our own sake, we must answer them for the sake of those who love us and who don't deserve the heartache of doubt after the first heartache of their loss.

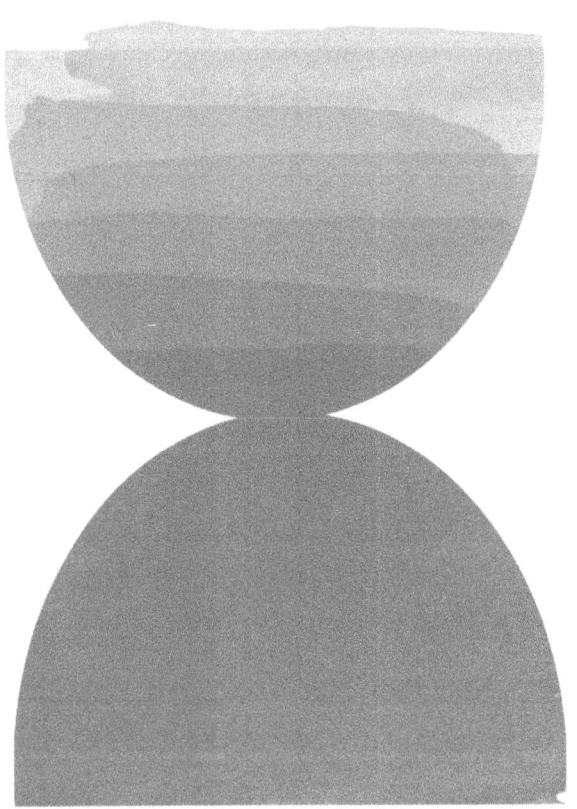

The pros and cons of clinical trials

Dum spiro, spero.
While I breathe, I hope.
Saint Andrew

CLINICAL TRIALS may seem an odd thing to mention in a book about dying well, but judging by the number of people I meet who hold out hope for a trial before dying, they are worth discussing. While we commonly hear of clinical trials in the context of cancer, they exist for all sorts of conditions – from insomnia and migraines to diabetes and stroke. Doctors suggest enrolling in a clinical trial when conventional options don't exist or have been exhausted. Trials are also used to study therapies that have shown promise in the lab but require more evidence before being approved for common use.

It was through clinical trials that we learnt about the importance of administering aspirin during a heart attack and how to limit brain damage after a stroke. It's how we got better at treating asthma, anaphylaxis and diabetes and how we found that strong drugs like morphine cause more harm than good in conditions such as chronic back pain.

Clinical trials have also shown us that drugs cannot reverse dementia, antibiotics don't work against viruses, the removal of a cancerous breast lump is as effective as a mastectomy and some cases of appendicitis can be managed without an operation. In my own field of oncology, there isn't a week that goes by without the report of a promising clinical trial to ease the burden of cancer sufferers.

The knowledge gained from clinical trials betters millions of lives, which is why doctors, advocacy organisations and patients clamour for access to trials. Indeed, we ought to be indebted to all trial participants for advancing the cause of patients all over the world.

However, the fact is that less than five per cent of the patient population enrols in trials and most seriously ill people or those at the end of life are ineligible due to stringent qualifying criteria, geographical location, or other intensive logistics. Yet I can't help but notice that the incentive to participate in a trial is never greater than when life is nearing its end and there is a deep urge to extend it. As an oncologist, I have a front seat to the phenomenon, and I believe that the lessons from patients enrolled in cancer clinical trials hold meaning for many of us.

First, a brief explanation.

Early-stage trials (Phase 1 and 2) run over several months to a few years and are designed to determine whether a drug is safe in humans, what dose works and what are the side effects. These trials establish basic knowledge about a drug, with approximately a third of early phase trials progressing to the next phase.

Late-stage (Phase 3) trials take several years to complete and study how the trial drug compares to the existing standard of care. Between a quarter to a third of drugs move to Phase 4, where the drug's safety and efficacy is monitored in volunteers who have the condition.

One way of accessing therapies not yet approved by regulatory bodies for widespread use is by enrolling in a clinical trial.

Medicine advances on the shoulders of trials. Participants usually gain the advantage of close monitoring and are the first to enjoy any benefits. It is gratifying to see patients with little option respond to an experimental therapy. Depending on the circumstances, some can remain well for a long time while others succumb to their illness quickly.

The evidence shows that there is poor understanding of the entire clinical trials process but especially the reason to enrol in one. Researchers take pains to explain that trials are fact-finding missions. The vast majority of drugs that appear promising in early-phase trials fail to get to market; less than five per cent are eventually approved. Late-phase trials don't help everyone gain quality or quantity of life. Participants might benefit but they're mainly laying the foundation for future patients by helping refine our understanding of disease.

Like most doctors who want to help their patients, I welcome the availability of clinical trials. Unfortunately, there is a gulf of understanding between what doctors know and what patients think. In my own experience, patients enrolling in clinical trials widely believe, or hope, that the trial drug will provide a cure, or at the very least meaningfully extend life. Consequently, when serious side effects erode quality of life, patients and their loved ones can feel very let down. Expectations gone awry can inject uncertainty into the dying process and make it more complicated.

Nisha worked at a grocery I used to frequent on my way to work. She'd cheerfully pick out the freshest produce for me as we exchanged hurried pleasantries. Nisha had great regard for my work because some of her friends were undergoing cancer treatment. I used to marvel at her ability to run a business and yet find the time to care deeply about the people in her life. When economics forced the closure of her shop, I missed our short chats. Years later, I was taken aback to see her on a hospital ward round. Her face lit up at our unexpected encounter but it took all my effort to suppress my alarm. Her gown half open to reveal her gaunt frame, she was struggling to manoeuvre her IV pole to get to the bathroom and collapsed at the edge of the bed to catch her breath. I could barely reconcile the image with that of the woman who used to greet me every morning.

I discovered that she'd been undergoing cancer treatment for two years at a different hospital. Her oncologist had put her on a 'last-ditch' drug, which kept making her sick; she was spending a lot of time in hospital, where blood transfusions and antibiotics did nothing.

Given the visible extent of illness and the poor progress she was describing, I knew she didn't have long to live. Clutching her side in discomfort, she said, 'But if this treatment doesn't work, I'm waiting to go on a clinical trial. And if they don't take me, I'll sell the house because I've heard good things about the drug.' With this, my dismay was complete.

I knew that she had a family who would never recover from the financial stress of funding a drug that was still undergoing testing. Nisha wasn't my patient, but I felt protective of her.

She asked me what I thought of her situation. Sitting down beside her, I replied truthfully that she looked unwell and that, before making any significant decisions, she should talk to her long-term oncologist. I couldn't imagine him recommending she sell the family home, but I also hoped that he'd broach the issue of her mortality, which she seemed unaware of.

The pros and cons of clinical trials

I gently proposed that sometimes the best option was to accept one's illness and focus on quality of life. In her case, this meant getting home with palliative care, having home oxygen, and adequate pain relief. She brightened at the thought of going home but felt helpless to make it happen.

'I'll probably die here.'

I promised to speak to her doctors and she thanked me.

As she held my hand, I couldn't help but notice hers, pockmarked by attempts at intravenous lines.

Afterwards, my day felt overcast as I mulled over things. How could Nisha feel helpless in the very system meant to help? How much responsibility lay with her oncologist who didn't want her to give up? Was she one of the 'fighters' who couldn't bear to face reality? Or did she have a family who believed that modern medicine had an antidote to every ill?

In all likelihood, it was a bit of each.

Not long afterwards, Nisha died. Overcome with sadness, I called her husband and learnt that she'd managed to get home for two weeks. Admiring her courage, he lamented her inability to have the trial drug. It felt ironic to reassure him that she'd never have qualified for a trial and that there was no evidence that the drug would've extended her life.

'Not even by a year or two?' he asked hopefully.

My heart sank at the wildly unrealistic estimation. Nisha had been looking to join a Phase 1 trial, the type that investigates whether a drug works at all. But his words were a testament to the desperation patients feel.

'I'm afraid not,' I replied, moved by the guilt he must have been harbouring.

Reflecting on how ill she'd been, he conceded that the last few months of her life would have been calmer had they known that she was dying. Despite being only fifty, she would have opted to stop treatment and cherish her time at home. His words were a reminder that when discussing the benefits and risks of a clinical trial, doctors must be constantly vigilant about discussing life expectancy.

While Nisha was dying, someone I knew with a rare autoimmune disease did manage to enrol in a clinical trial. Vince was an artist who saw his life being slowly compromised by severe fatigue, joint pain and reduced social engagement. After receiving just one dose of the experimental drug, he reported new symptoms. The next few doses exaggerated his troubles and the drug was stopped, but not before it left him with profound nerve damage, chronic pain and, worst of all, an inability to paint. As his outside interests were curtailed, painting had filled many empty hours, but now he could no longer hold a paintbrush.

A devastated Vince alleged that in the readiness to enrol him there had been a lack of informed consent about uncommon but serious toxicities. He thought that he had been given the fine print to read 'but the spoken emphasis was on the good outcomes'. Subsequently, deficient communication with the principal researcher had led to his complaints not being taken seriously.

He lodged a formal complaint and received a modest financial compensation. The researcher was reprimanded, and the trial governance was strengthened. Vince died shortly afterwards, having lost his zest for life.

Vince's story is not an argument against clinical trial participation but a reminder to understand our options fully and not hesitate to ask questions.

In recent times, a prominent Australian trial was retracted by the *Journal of the American Medical Association*, a full two years after publication, when it emerged that the principal researcher had concocted patients and fabricated data about a common blood pressure drug. Given the high prevalence of cardiovascular disease, the impact of a positive study in a prestigious journal is substantial and wide-reaching and this finding was quoted more than thirty times. Many doctors read the original conclusion and changed the way they managed patients but failed to see the retraction.

The story of promising trial results being retracted or unable to be replicated is all too common. Notorious retracted studies include one that claimed a link between the measles vaccine and autism, whose ripple effect continues to harm children who are not vaccinated. The author of an influential study on human cloning and stem cells was found dead soon after his findings were debunked as fabricated. Other fraudulent researchers have been barred from government funding, sometimes decades after their actions.

Most patients and doctors are unaware of the ugly underbelly of clinical trials, the practice of unscrupulous researchers and large pharmaceutical companies prioritising sales over patient welfare. Upstanding scientists rightly bristle at this broad generalisation and point out the greater good from well-conducted trials which advance the cause of all patients, but there is truth to both sides.

Finally, there is another important but invisible aspect of clinical trials that should matter to everyone: deception by volunteers who participate in paid studies. In a recent finding, a quarter of volunteers exaggerated their symptoms to qualify for a paid study and fourteen percent pretended to have a health condition in order to join the study. The latter would be difficult in the case of cancer but less so in trials studying pain, fatigue or anxiety.

By falsifying their account, participants undermine the integrity of the entire study by biasing the data. Whether a trial is studying the value of a test or the toxicity of a drug, participants who report their experience with anything less than total honesty can substantially alter findings, leading to the discontinuation of a valuable trial or conversely, continuation of an unsafe one. Serious toxicity can be attributed to the experimental medication when the culprit is an illicit drug or a drug interaction. Alternatively, a drug trial that mistakenly includes patients suffering from a given condition instead of healthy volunteers may be biased in favour of the drug.

Despite some of the obstacles associated with clinical trials, evidence is our best friend when it comes to selecting the most appropriate painkiller, the best chemotherapy, or the safest surgical technique.

Before recommending a clinical trial, doctors must consider if it is the right move for their most seriously ill patients. We must apply a ceaselessly enquiring mind to the reams of data thrust upon us every day and not be afraid to acknowledge that in many areas of medicine, there is no one right answer. Importantly, for patients, it means having a curious mind and being unafraid to ask questions. With the power imbalance between doctors and patients this isn't easy but, more than ever, it's necessary. Ironically, sometimes being ineligible for a trial provides the closure someone needs.

It's human nature to want to explore every possible avenue of hope. When it comes to searching for a clinical trial towards the end of life, these considerations take on profound meaning. The stakes are higher when time is limited – many of us desire to cherish our time with family and friends but some people find satisfaction from pursuing treatments until the end of life. As long as we are fully informed, it is for each of us to decide what matters most.

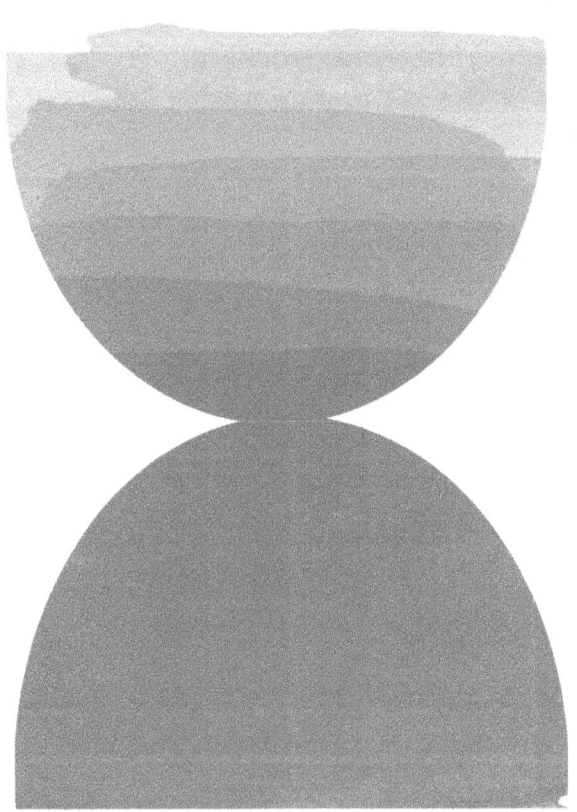

Protecting our health

The first wealth is health.
Ralph Waldo Emerson

Twenty years of experience in medicine has taught me that dying well has a necessary precedent, living well. And while living well doesn't guarantee a good death, it definitely helps to guard against some of the complications that befall those who suffer from the so-called 'lifestyle' diseases that are on the rise.

I was quite fond of my patient Ron, who jokingly referred to himself as a couch potato although I could always sense his self-consciousness. Short and morbidly obese, Ron hated moving and loved to talk about his love of fat and sugar, preferably together. The first time we met he struggled to walk the short distance to my room before crashing into a chair and clutching its sides to regain his breath. I watched him with dismay because he was only in his mid-fifties.

I'd told Ron when I met him that his cancer was inoperable but there was a good chance of inducing a remission with chemotherapy. However, I knew that his poor fitness would hamper his ability to cope with intensive therapy.

Patients with obesity, uncontrolled diabetes, poor cardiovascular fitness, excessive alcohol and cigarette consumption and other chronic diseases experience a significantly higher risk of complications and death. Even ordinary setbacks take on heavy meaning and it can be extremely challenging to guide such patients back to health.

Ron joked that he'd try not to be my 'nightmare' patient but his wife, Sue, looked worried. One week before starting chemotherapy, Ron developed pneumonia. He responded to antibiotics but even I was surprised by how quickly he became deconditioned. The effort of walking to the bathroom exhausted him and he needed a hand to get out of bed. Sent to rehabilitation, he developed a urinary tract infection there and nearly died from sepsis. But he rallied and must have seen the relief written all over my face. When every week mattered, there was no room for delay.

With a marathon effort, Ron got home, began chemotherapy, and survived the first month. But just as I relaxed, he landed in hospital with a bowel obstruction and I dreaded what would surely follow. He was prescribed pain relief and started on artificial nutrition to help rest his bowel, but his poor general health meant he had no reserve left.

Some days later, his surgeon called me to share her dilemma over the obstinate bowel obstruction. She felt he would die without an operation but had an equal risk of dying as a result of the operation. The decision about what to do had to involve us all and, most of all, the deteriorating patient.

Despite his obvious unwellness, I was touched by Ron's usual good humour. People kept entering his room to adjust his intravenous lines, monitor his vital signs and check on his comfort – he raised his hand to acknowledge each one. I sat down next to him and told him we needed to talk. Drawing a picture to illustrate his predicament, I told him I'd understand his decision to have surgery but would support him unequivocally if he chose to avoid surgery and be palliated. No matter how many times I have this conversation, it never feels easy, but by now I have learnt its value.

Ron decided to take a chance at surgery. He hugged me for supporting him and I felt glum at our last good exchange. I couldn't help thinking of his surgeon and the emotional toll of such a risky undertaking for the entire surgical team.

Thanks to modern anaesthetics and a skilled team, Ron's blockage was cleared and he survived the surgery. However, he developed another infection and this time failed to regain consciousness. Three days later, with the writing on the wall, his heartbroken wife made the decision to withdraw intensive care. I visited Ron with enormous regret shortly before he died. His many tubes had been removed and the machines surrounding him had fallen silent. He looked grey and had suddenly aged many years, but flanked by his family, I thought he appeared more restful than in all the time I had known him.

While the ultimate cause of Ron's death was cancer, his dismal state of fitness had caused his untimely death. Not for the first time, I thought about how little people understand the deadly impact of the benign-sounding term 'lifestyle factors'.

A growing body of evidence supports the role of lifestyle modifications in preventing chronic illness. For instance, reflecting on the untold grief and heartache that cancer causes, researchers recently found that that even small improvements in our lifestyle have the potential to translate into important health gains. Nearly forty per cent of cancers are thought to be preventable. Of course, there are many other causes of ill health we ought to be concerned about, not only cancer. Silent diseases that shorten our lives and that the majority of us will experience, either for ourselves or through our loved ones, include heart disease, diabetes, organ failure and dementia.

Some lifestyle risk factors are modifiable, which means we can reduce our personal risk, and others are fixed, such as age, gender, race and family history. We have the power to reduce the risk of developing chronic disease by making better dietary choices, eating a little less, moving a little more, not smoking, curbing alcohol and maintaining a healthy weight. Fostering close relationships and safeguarding our emotional health are other important aspects of living well. All this might make for a tough prescription, but health clinics and hospitals are overflowing with people who face the serious impact of having neglected their health.

In hospitals that are the seat of so much bad news, one instantly uplifting thing is to meet ninety-year-old patients – and even some centenarians – in better health than people half their age. Doctors and nurses marvel at their well-being and good-naturedly enquire about their secret. I note some broad attributes in such patients: they have usually avoided smoking, used alcohol with restraint, and have maintained a healthy weight through a balanced diet and exercise. They've adjusted their expectations with age, remained socially engaged and found a different purpose with passing years. This contentment is infectious. When their health deteriorates, many die peacefully and their loved ones describe a quiet sense of closure. Of course, not every death is the same and there can be surprise, grief and controversy at all ages. But being a doctor at the end of life is to be reminded of the relationship between living well and dying peacefully.

We cannot control every aspect of our life but on top of our list ought to be our physical health and emotional well-being. Our death may be inevitable, but we have a role in making our lives better and longer. There are abundant guidelines on weight management, safe alcohol consumption and how to stop smoking, and many of us have access to public space for exercise. These changes need not be expensive or complicated, or require a professional; they simply require us to acknowledge that the cost of making these changes pales in comparison to that of dealing with a chronically poor quality of life.

We all know people who pledge to change their behaviour in response to a wake-up call. It's far better to benefit from the experience of others and protect our health from the outset. As an old saying goes, he who has health has hope; he who has hope has everything.

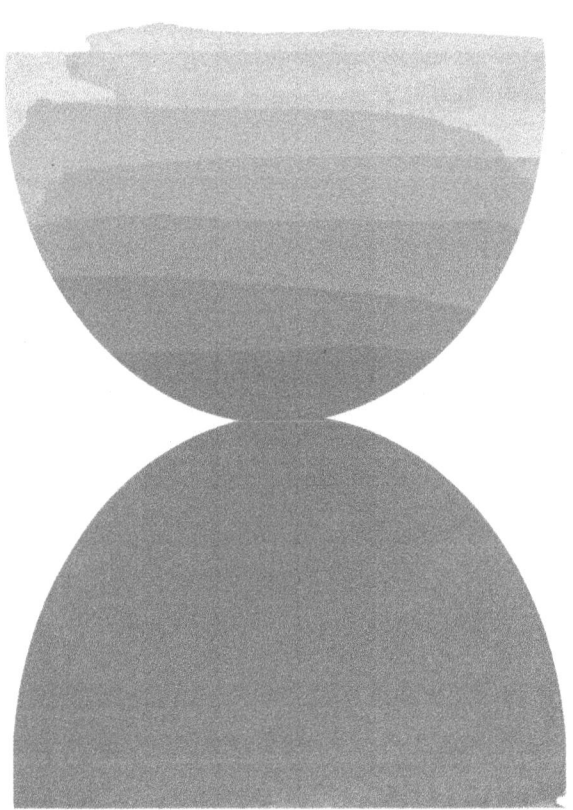

Tackling pain at the end of life

Do not mock a pain you have not endured.
The Quran

'So, you're saying there is nothing you can do.'

'That's not what I said,' I gently reminded Milos. 'Chemotherapy will be harmful, but I want to treat your pain.'

'But without chemo, I'll die.'

Perhaps the most common conversation I have with patients in the last phase of their life is whether forgoing treatment equates to giving up, and hence inviting premature death. In fact, this couldn't be further from the truth. In most cases, aggressive interventions at the end of life are known to do more harm than good and can lead to a poorer quality of life and potentially reduced survival.

'I'm afraid you're too unwell for chemotherapy, though reducing your pain is a good goal.'

At eighty-eight, Milos was frail and worn-out merely from the effort of walking to my room. Small-statured, bony and painfully thin, it seemed a gust of wind might tilt his balance were it not for his sturdy walking frame. He was so desperate to have more treatment that I felt I had but one chance to convince him otherwise. It's easy to extinguish the flickering hope of dying patients but it will never be more important to care about their holistic needs.

As he looked at me sceptically, I feared I'd lost. I watched him squirming in his chair, brusquely downplaying his pain, noticing how people tried to disguise their discomfort to protect their loved ones and present their best side to the doctor.

His daughter looked upset, having seen his desperation and sensed my caution. She explained that he couldn't fathom having an incurable illness and I sympathised that, while I couldn't alter its prognosis, I could confidently ease his symptoms.

'Let me prescribe you a small dose of morphine,' I suggested.

He recoiled in horror. 'Oh no, I'm not touching morphine!'

His daughter's face filled with consternation, as if the mention of morphine had made the news even worse.

I reassured them that morphine and related opioids weren't simply used at the very end of life; they could also ease pain and improve quality of life, helping people function better.

At this, Milos fretted that he didn't want to become an 'addict' and I quickly moved to dismantle a misconception that might compromise his eventual end-of-life care.

I differentiated opioid abuse from its judicious use to relieve severe pain. He listened attentively but without conviction, so I left the door open for discussion and his daughter agreed to update me. Just days later, she rang a nurse to explain that Milos was at crisis point and, this time, too despondent and fed up to protest at having morphine.

Within two days, his pain had receded, and he was sleeping without interruption, reducing his irritability and improving his appetite. Relief from the constant pain of the past several weeks made for lucid thoughts and he accepted a home visit from palliative care. I was gratified to note that a patient who had until recently disavowed all supports quickly accepted all advocacy. The palliative care team monitored his comfort, counselled his wife, and became a reassuring presence in the family's life. On subsequent hospital visits, Milos never referred to chemotherapy again but often mentioned his gratitude at being largely free of pain.

His situation fragile but stable, Milos could venture into his garden, which lifted his spirits. His wife was especially happy at this and I found myself thinking that no other treatment could have brought greater relief than a small dose of morphine. This is why the World Health Organisation lists morphine on the essential drugs list for end-of-life care.

As his illness advanced, so did the need for higher doses of morphine, which created the added effects of constipation and drowsiness. But knowing what to expect made it easier to deal with these symptoms.

Milos lived for three months after his diagnosis. He died comfortably, surrounded by his wife, children and grandchildren, as he had hoped.

———

PAIN IS A UNIVERSALLY FEARED SYMPTOM at the end of life. Many people find the courage to ask if they will experience pain, others worry but are too afraid to say anything. This is why I believe that professionals have a duty to specifically address it and caregivers must be attuned to pain.

I reassure my patients that there are many ways to relieve pain, depending on its location, frequency and available resources. Unfortunately, large parts of the world lack access to pain relief but, elsewhere too, pain relief is often hampered by a lack of recognition, deficient expertise and widely prevalent misconceptions. As someone who prescribes opioids nearly every day, I have acquired a healthy respect for their efficacy as well as their dangers. Here are some practical tips everyone should know.

Opioids shouldn't be vilified. Morphine is virtually irreplaceable in situations of severe burns, postoperative recovery, cancer pain and palliative care but there is good evidence that it provides no additional benefit over simple drugs like paracetamol and ibuprofen when taken for migraines, back pain, arthritis and other conditions associated with chronic pain. The opioid epidemic has been fuelled by the inappropriate use of opioids, which researchers now recognise can worsen the experience of pain and even prove fatal. When it comes to dying with comfort, however, morphine can be invaluable.

Some of my terminally ill patients report being allergic to morphine. On closer questioning, they have usually experienced nausea, vomiting or drowsiness after taking the drug in an emergency or after surgery.

These symptoms rarely point to a true allergy and may not be necessarily related to the drug. Since morphine can make an indisputable difference to quality of life, it's important for patients to recall a thorough history of morphine use. Now that opioids are available in many different types and formulations, it's almost always possible to help patients derive their benefit while being spared the side effects. The need for painkillers can fluctuate and many people must try different opioids before finding one that suits. It's also important to ensure a sufficient supply of opioids to avoid the stress of suddenly running out and a relationship with the family doctor is important in ensuring up-to-date scripts.

Finally, there is no 'best' opioid – ultimately what matters is taking a drug that works, is safe, and provides a sense of control.

Pain relief is an inexact science and an area of medicine that suffers from underinvestment. As a specialty it has gained prominence only in the last few decades; consequently, many doctors have the intention but not the training to help their most complex patients including those at the end of life. But since pain can be so onerous, distressing and disabling, we all deserve better.

While physical pain is evident, there is a category of pain even harder to treat: existential distress.

Uncertainty, anxiety and depression at the end of life are common and have a detrimental effect on patients and their caregivers. Patients with unresolved existential distress frequently experience reduced trust in their doctor, which makes it difficult for them to share their deepest concerns. Prolonged lack of engagement can lead to a poor end-of-life experience.

We all have a role to play in recognising and managing existential distress as it is an important part of dying well. Individual therapy, group counselling, cognitive behavioural therapy and, in some instances, prescription medication play a role in alleviating emotional distress.

We might wonder if the prospect of death isn't naturally depressing for everyone but I've learnt this isn't true. Many dying patients, young and old, express satisfaction with the life they have led and have reconciled to the things they were unable to do. They have accepted their mortality as an inalterable fact of life; instead of begrudging the inevitable, they've slowed down and focused on making the most of their time. This has buoyed their spirits and aided others in the journey.

Pain – physical or existential – does not have to be unquestionable or untreatable. We deserve to die with dignity and comfort and should never be afraid to demand this for ourselves and our loved ones.

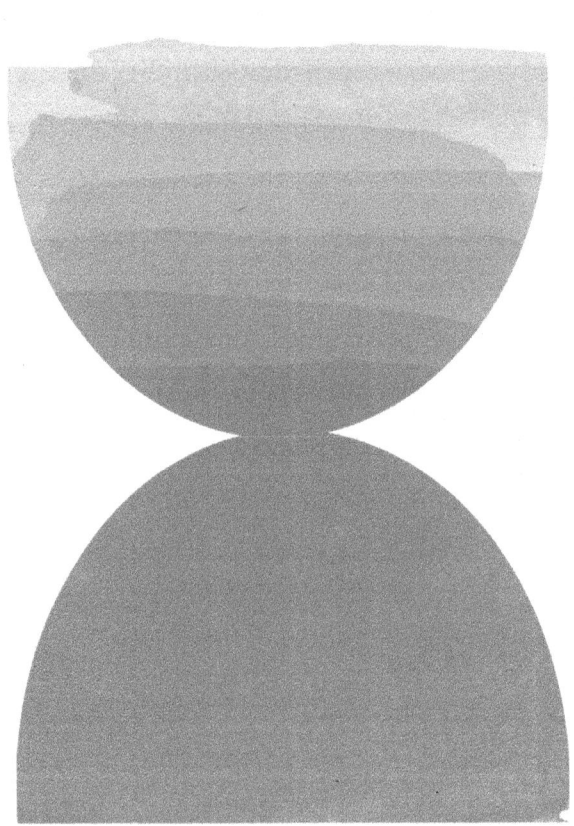

What to do about denial

*For life and death are one even as the
river and sea are one.*

Khalil Gibran

I HAD HEARD MANY STORIES about denial, but received my first taste of it when a patient lodged a complaint about me for telling her the truth that she had demanded to know about her terminal illness. Her complaint rattled my confidence and left me questioning the duty of a doctor ever since.

Julia was a woman in her fifties, diagnosed with advanced lung cancer at a time when there were few good treatments. The chemotherapy prescribed by her oncologist had helped her briefly but now she was in hospital with a serious complication of her disease known as spinal cord compression. She had been experiencing several days of leg weakness and stumbling, but when she suddenly became incontinent, she was alarmed.

Scans found extensive tumour pressing on her spinal cord, the control centre of the nervous system. The tumour was inoperable and it was doubtful that any other treatment would reverse the progressive paralysis that had developed from her waist down.

I met Julia for the first time the morning after the tests. One of the hardest situations for any doctor is to reveal bad news at the first encounter. But the worse the news the greater the imperative for disclosure – patients deserve to know the truth.

Introducing myself as an oncologist, I asked if she had pain.

'I'm comfortable,' she replied, 'but I'd really like to know how long I've got.'

Everyone agrees that, ideally, this conversation is best had with a doctor who has a history with the patient, who has travelled the ups and downs and knows not only the course of the illness but the social and emotional context within which the illness has unfolded. But her oncologist wasn't prepared to travel for what he deemed a foreseeable complication of her condition. He didn't offer to speak to Julia, didn't return her calls and she was in no fit state to travel to him. It was frustrating, but I confined myself to helping Julia rather than guessing at her oncologist's motivations.

Dr Ranjana Srivastava

Cancer patients with spinal cord compression are among those with the poorest prognosis. Due to the lack of movement or sensation in her legs, Julia was confined to bed and had the beginnings of pneumonia. Any infection involving her already compromised lungs did not bode well.

I silently took stock of all the news I needed to convey to Julia, and her husband, Hugh, to help them make decisions in her best interest. When we met, they seemed prepared to hear the bad news they'd probably been expecting since her diagnosis. I had started explaining the futility of further chemotherapy when Julia interrupted: 'Can you tell me if I will live until Christmas?'

I remember gazing outside at the crisp June morning at the usual rush of cars and pedestrians in front of the hospital. Did Julia have another six months to live? Would she recover from this catastrophe and be like one of the other patients I could spot going in and out of the hospital?

My heart said please, let it be so, but my gut instinct said no. Doctors aren't soothsayers and one of the most humbling things about medicine is how often we get things wrong but, based on the evidence before me, I had to let Julia know what I thought.

So I told her that while I hoped she'd prove me wrong, I couldn't be sure she would survive until Christmas and consequently, we should discuss her goals. Julia frowned, and I held my breath at the revelation of a birth or wedding or some immovable event. But she said her main aim was to organise Christmas gifts for her three adult children and plan a lunch with her extended family. This was achievable and, for the next half hour, we discussed how to prepare for what lay ahead. She mentioned writing notes and calling her friends. Hugh wanted to take her away. They both agreed to meet the palliative care nurse. In fact, our conversation took on such a positive energy that I was impressed by the couple's resilience under the most testing circumstances.

As I left, Julia and Hugh thanked me tearfully for the most honest and helpful conversation they'd had during her entire illness; one that would now help inform several important decisions. Undeserving as I felt of their praise, I couldn't have asked for a better outcome.

So, nothing could have prepared me for the reception next morning when a senior nurse approached me to say that, hours after our conversation, Julia had filed a complaint about my conduct, alleging that I had inflicted extreme distress on the entire family by discussing her prognosis. I was dumbfounded.

The nurse reflected that Julia was in denial and best given some privacy although the irony didn't escape me that the nurse had chosen to stop me in the middle of the busiest thoroughfare where I was surrounded by medical students and residents, all of whom had witnessed my indictment.

Dr Ranjana Srivastava

Despite my roiling sentiments, my first instinct was to apologise to Julia, thinking that the antidote to her vehement reaction was to approach her with kindness. But to my horror, Julia had banned me from her bedside. My humiliation felt complete but, putting on a brave face, I told my team that such setbacks were part of one's career and they shouldn't dissuade us from doing the right thing.

Not only did Julia refuse to see me but she also turned away other doctors and discharged herself from hospital. I discovered later that she'd apparently never understood from her oncologist that she had a terminal illness, although he refuted this.

Julia's public outburst prompted widespread dismay and soul-searching amongst professionals. A nurse who'd witnessed my exchange with Julia and Hugh consoled me that I'd done nothing wrong. A junior doctor said she'd lost the courage to raise such a sensitive subject with the next patient. I kept replaying the scene in my mind, wondering what I could have done differently.

The palliative care team stepped in to help, but she was determined to prove everyone wrong. Out of respect, I didn't contact Julia again, but I heard that she died within some weeks of going home. It must have been a particularly difficult time for Hugh and her children, who had to manage on their own.

Many years on, I remember the incident as if it happened yesterday. I hate to think that my words were ultimately responsible for a patient's suffering and a family's consternation and even now the prospect of a family meeting to discuss prognosis makes me pause.

Every year I meet a few extremely ill patients engaged in circular conversations about their mortality. They can't believe there's no reasonable treatment left for their illness and insist on a solution. Multiple family conferences explore their deterioration but fail to produce insights. These patients are exhausted in body but resistant in their mind. Consequently, many feel chronically dissatisfied and restless, waiting for medicine to propose a solution.

Denial at the end of life is a problem that impacts everyone who encounters it. It's said to arise from misinformation, misunderstanding and a lack of communication between doctors and patients. All this is true, but my experience of patients in denial have taught me something else. With enough humility and insight, the errors of communication can be corrected, information gaps can be plugged and understanding reached. But what no one can touch is the resolute denial that resides within people, and which refuses to acknowledge that we are all mortal. This type of denial involves fear, sadness and panic, but at its core is a failure to have thought about life as a gift – and an ephemeral one at that. Helping people overcome denial is the most challenging aspect of caring for the dying.

Dr Ranjana Srivastava

It's instructive being a doctor to these patients. While they are hard to satisfy, the challenges their professionals face pale in comparison to the stress endured by their loved ones. Their caregivers deserve sympathy because, although they might appreciate the truth, they are frequently reduced to being hapless bystanders. It takes great patience and love to look beyond their frustrations and accord the individual dignity and respect.

What I have learnt is that strong denial never goes away in one grand leap of realisation. Instead, it requires a series of small steps.

Many times, denial dissipates as a patient confronts unavoidable realities such as growing fatigue and disability. But sometimes, denial actually demands graceful acceptance on the part of the rest of us. We don't stop caring but we stop feeling bad about the situation.

Medicine has a long way to go towards helping patients in denial. But I can't help thinking that ultimately this is a task that belongs intimately to every one of us. It's never too early to learn that we have a limited life in which to give and receive. A child needs to know why a grandparent is dying. An adolescent must make sense of the death of a parent. When elders bury their young, and the natural order of things feels disrupted, we should mourn with them but also acknowledge the universality of death. This is how all of us, young and old, can accept our mortality.

Confucius said that we have two lives, the second of which begins when we realise we only have one. Two thousand years later psychiatrist Elisabeth Kübler-Ross reflected that 'It is the denial of death that is partially responsible for people living empty, purposeless lives; for when you live as if you'll live forever, it becomes too easy to postpone the things you know that you must do.'

Perhaps it's by blending ancient wisdom with modern perspective that each one of us can define for ourselves what it means to live well and die well.

Dr Ranjana Srivastava

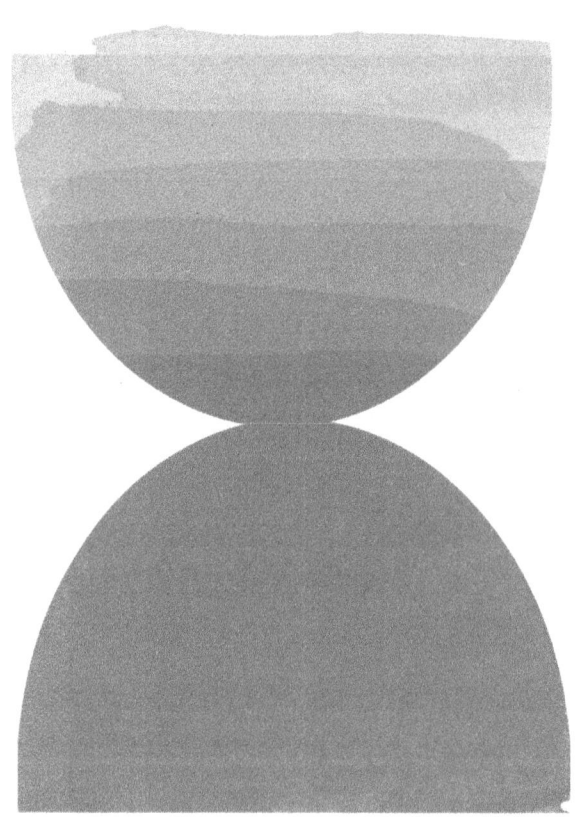

Dealing with a sudden death

Let us endeavour so to live that when we come to die even the undertaker will be sorry.

Mark Twain

BEING AN INTERN for a year in a large hospital is a lesson in hard work performed in virtual anonymity. An intern is expected to quietly follow the rules, avoid controversy and generally shun the limelight. Like all interns, I became used to being at the back of the herd of doctors at the bedside each day, dutifully recording the specialist's instructions. Busy specialists operate through a hierarchy: they mainly talk to the fellow, who briefs the senior resident, who manages the junior resident, who works with the intern. An intern may have very little direct communication with the specialist and being so far removed from the real decision-making can be an almost innocuous experience were it not for the responsibility one feels as even the most junior member of the team.

That's why I nearly jumped out of my skin when, the next year, I became a junior resident and was assigned to work with a prominent specialist who greeted me by my full name and shook my hand. While I furiously searched my brain for a reason he would know me, he pleasantly reminded me that we had met when I had dropped in to see patients in the intensive care unit where he worked. He always remembered names, he said. He sounded genuine, but I was dubious that he could file away hundreds of names and associations just like that.

But Ramesh would soon prove me wrong. On one of our first medical ward rounds together, an elderly, sleep-deprived patient was so startled by our presence that she dropped her orange juice, which bounced off her tray and landed on the floor, but not before collecting Ramesh's pressed suit.

The other doctors reflexively jumped out of the way but he calmly retrieved the empty tub, reassured the mortified patient, alerted the cleaner and continued the round without missing a beat. Some hours later, I returned to write my notes and found the cleaner at the desk. With tears in her eyes, she related that in twenty years, many specialists had summoned her help, but none had known her name.

'It's because no one thinks I'm important.'

Dr Ranjana Srivastava

Her remark is etched in my memory because I think she was right.

Ramesh turned out to be one of the nicest doctors I ever worked with. He was blessed with erudition and etiquette. In a deep and sonorous voice that had once graced the cricket commentary, he conducted bedside and teaching rounds that left a mark on doctors and patients. In matters of respect and collegiality, he didn't distinguish between a top surgeon and a student nurse; in conversation, he could skilfully explain a concept to a puzzled patient and provide a scientific explanation to the keen doctor. To those who knew him, he epitomised good medicine.

Ramesh was an intensive care specialist and I was training to become an oncologist, leading to a professional parting, and it would have been rather easy to lose touch had he not been an early and enthusiastic advocate of my writings on the intersection of humanity with medicine. A great believer in compassion and empathy in dealings with patients, he was frequently found debating the meaning of medicine with young doctors. He also wrote eloquently, so as I embarked on my writing career, few things brought me more joy than a handwritten note from him.

Ramesh mentored me through my early years of training, saw me become an oncologist, consoled me when I lost a late-term twin pregnancy, celebrated my newborn children, read my early drafts, commended my books, and invited me to speak about the art of medicine at the conferences he organised. He once told me that his favorite part of the conference was watching young doctors prosper, as it meant his job was done. But I think for many in the audience, the most memorable part of every conference was the tribute he insisted on paying the hard-working kitchen staff, who were brought out to a standing ovation. This was a man who saw the best in everyone.

In an all-consuming career, Ramesh was fortunate to have an extremely capable and patient wife who'd willingly given up her own career in medicine to support their children. As we became busier, Ramesh and I spoke and emailed more than we met. In his early fifties, he felt pulled in many directions but was beginning to realise the need to slow down and spend more time at home.

I had just finished seeing the last patient of the morning, a pleasant eighty-year-old man who'd recovered well from surgery and left me thinking gladly about some of the wonders of modern medicine, when there was a knock on my door. A doctor had dropped in to say hello.

'You don't know?' he asked

'Know what?'

'Ramesh died an hour ago.'

I thought I'd misheard him, or he was talking about someone I didn't know.

'What did you say?'

'Ramesh suffered a cardiac arrest this morning and couldn't be revived.'

Looking at the disbelief on my face, the poor doctor added, 'I'm really sorry, I thought you'd be one of the first to know.'

But I was still reeling from the news. An arrest, yes, but had Ramesh actually died? Perhaps people were still working on him.

'Is it a rumour?'

'No, I spoke to a doctor who was there. He couldn't be saved.'

I took a deep breath to calm myself and declared that I had to see Ramesh myself.

My hands were on the steering wheel, but my mind felt numb as I mechanically drove the familiar route. Reaching the hospital, I rushed to the cardiac unit and spotted his wife standing forlornly outside a single room.

Ramesh's body lay on a narrow white bed, his expression as serene as if he were asleep. His hands felt warm, his complexion had yet to take on the greyness of death. There was not a single sign of the grim fight to keep him alive, involving every expert at hand. I sat beside him, robbed of speech and thought, just one word ricocheting in my head: 'Why?'

Aware of the health risks of a middle-aged man, he had undergone a normal cardiac workup just weeks ago. That morning, he had been getting ready for work when he experienced mild chest pain. Reassured by his recent health clearance, he nevertheless decided to get checked. His wife offered to take him to the nearby hospital where he was scheduled to work.

They assumed he'd be fine and conduct his ward round there but what happened next would turn into a recurring nightmare.

Nearly at the hospital, Ramesh slumped in his seat. His doctor wife had to make the unenviable decision between stopping on the freeway and driving another few minutes, and decided to keep driving. Minutes later, the emergency department leapt into action and experts flooded in to try every known intervention. But according to the person whose hands ached from performing prolonged chest compressions, Ramesh had sustained such a massive cardiac arrest that he never had a chance. Following three hours of non-stop effort and an unimaginably emotional ordeal, the very doctors who called Ramesh a colleague and friend had to admit defeat and pronounce him dead. The people preparing to do a round with him that morning had to make room for his lifeless body, write his death certificate, and still carry on with the work of looking after their other patients. That day and the ensuing days and weeks would be some of their worst. As for the family, their trauma had just begun.

Dr Ranjana Srivastava

As an oncologist, I'm used to caring for patients who slowly decline and die. There's time to grieve, adjust and anticipate. Sudden death provides none of these consolations. Unfortunately, over the years, I have witnessed many such deaths too, a few from catastrophic illness but more commonly due to accidents and suicide. The high rates of burnout, substance abuse and mental illness in the medical profession mean that many doctors know someone who has succumbed to a drug overdose or committed suicide. I have lost colleagues without having an inkling that there was something wrong with them – interns who didn't show up to work; specialists at the peak of their career; nurses who ran a ward just a week earlier.

I've also lost patients who were not expected to die just yet. We reassured them that they were on the mend and told their families to go home for the night. Then something unpredictable happened. The patient suffered a heart attack, stopped breathing, or simply failed to wake up for lunch.

Once, mid-conversation on a ward round, I drew back the curtains to find a deceased elderly patient. His nurse had just set down his cup of tea and had gone to ready the shower. We all needed a few minutes to process our shock.

And like so many others, I have mourned family members with whom I shared a meal one night and whose funeral I attended later that week. Relatives I assumed I would grow old with but who died without notice. It seems hardly fair that death could be so brisk and remorseless and yet, as many of us will experience, it is exactly so.

In the grip of grief, people often wonder which is better, an expected death or a sudden one, as if we could ever settle our views on this perennial question.

However, having witnessed many deaths and discussed the aftermath with others, I can share my observations.

An expected death, predicted to the extent that it can be, provides an opportunity for conversations, with ourselves and those near and dear to us. These conversations can be practical – how we wish to divide our property, who should receive our jewellery, and how we want to wrap up our business – to the philosophical: who we should thank, who we must ask for forgiveness, and which of our beliefs and gestures will console us in the end. For loved ones, an anticipated death allows a final chance to understand people and honour their final wishes.

While this presents a rich opportunity to tie the loose ends of our mortal life and set the conditions for dying well, it would be a stretch to say this is indeed how most people die. From what I see, many of us die clinging to hope, reluctant to reconcile to our mortality, our affairs unsorted not unlike our wardrobe, unable to affirm what really matters. The heaviest consequence is that we let other people, including doctors, make significant decisions on our behalf without knowing us. Therefore, an opportunity to die well doesn't mean we actually die well – something that deserves thinking about.

As I have seen for myself, sudden death is instantaneously shattering and very traumatic. The grief may not be greater but there has been no time to gather our coping skills.

One day, I was crossing a busy road and thinking about my next meeting when a friend called me about our colleague's suicide – I'd recently waved to him in the corridor. Another time, my plane had just touched the tarmac when a text message flashed on my screen: a young woman I'd had dinner with the previous night had died.

It's hard to not be blown away by the sheer relentlessness of an event that gives no warning that a meal, a hug, a walk, or an argument might be our last. The kind of death that makes no room for prior realisation or reconciliation. That may come later, but first we will have to contend with our unexpected loss and the churning thoughts about what we could have done differently.

The person who loses a loved one slowly wishes to avoid a lingering death. The loved one mourning a sudden death pleads for more time. No matter how people die, death stings.

According to a fable, a king once asked some wise men to come up with a saying that would hold true in good times and bad. After deliberating, they handed him a ring that had etched on its inside, *This too shall pass.* My most admirable patients live by this dictum, knowing that to live wisely is to meet both joy and sorrow with equanimity. This realisation gives meaning to their lives and forges a legacy in their wake. It doesn't hasten their death; instead, it renders their remaining life more pleasurable.

But how should we prepare ourselves and our loved ones for our own death, sudden or otherwise? I can't help thinking that Ramesh led the kind of life that made it easier for people to move forward.

In the days after he died, there was a roaring silence on the wards and people went out of their way to avoid each other so as not to be reminded of their lost colleague. The wound felt deep and penetrating and insufferable. And to be honest, unfair. How could an octogenarian golfer survive a heart attack but not someone much younger? What could we do to protect our loved ones from such a fate?

In the years since his death, it's been instructive to watch the healing process and relate much of it to how Ramesh conducted himself in life.

His kindness and concern for others meant there was a groundswell of support to commemorate him. His colleagues continued an annual conference in his name and young doctors were moved to give back to others as he had done for them.

Dr Ranjana Srivastava

This created a community of mourners instead of helpless individuals.

His wife, blessed with an innate calm, was left in an unimaginably difficult situation to care for their two children. She made a conscious decision to not lament her fate but be grateful for the years they had together and remember the good he brought to the lives of others. I can't help thinking that she was greatly helped by the genuine respect and grief for Ramesh that reached her from far-flung corners of the world. Having been largely insulated from his professional life, she was consoled that her sacrifices had been for a greater cause.

On the subject of what we can do to help loved ones grieving a sudden death, there's actually a great deal that doesn't need undue effort. One is overcoming our own sense of shock or betrayal and reaching out to someone, a profoundly therapeutic act.

The weeks after my colleague's suicide were very challenging for all those who knew him. He was funny, talented, and enormously popular – it made no sense that he didn't appreciate this. Some doctors attended a memorial, others sought counselling, some were desperate for details, while others wrestled with conflicting emotions. Some of his closest friends were angry and confused. We had to accept our different reactions and it took time to recover, although he is still missed.

I attended every function held in Ramesh's honour and also gave the eulogy. It was one of the hardest things I've done. Sometime later, I visited his wife, unsure of what to say and never having imagined such an occasion. She showed me a mountain of cards she'd received, so we sat in companionable silence, reading the recollections and condolences of all the people he had touched. I remember thinking how deeply consoling it felt that Ramesh's loss was also felt by others. Indeed, a sorrow shared was a sorrow divided. I have never since underestimated the power of a thoughtful card or a short visit as a mark of care and respect for the deceased and those who survive.

In the course of my work I meet many relatives who dread the death of a loved one and say they couldn't possibly go on. But in truth, they find out that we humans have a tremendous capacity for resilience and recovery. We may not have thought of an alternative plan for life when things are working but, when circumstances demand it, we find a way because we are profoundly adaptable. We should take heart from this.

Which brings us back to living well even when the choice of dying well is taken away from us. Whether we die an anticipated death, as most of us will, or die suddenly, our lifelong qualities are what we will be remembered by.

We should practise being content within ourselves and showing generosity in our dealings with others. We should mind our health and strive to live long and productive lives but behave as if our last days were upon us. To think and behave now as we intend to do at the end of our lives could help us craft a way to ease our own death and make it alright for others.

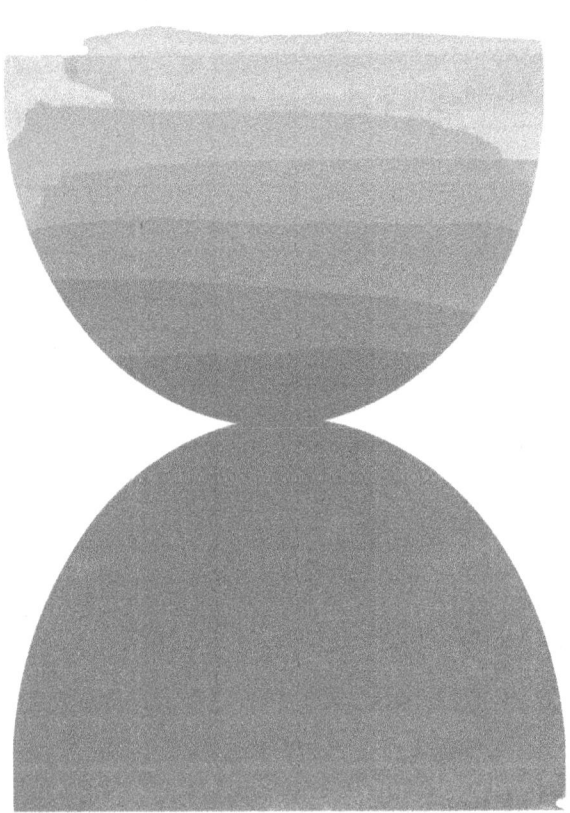

Facing the aftermath

To weep is to make less of the depth of grief.
William Shakespeare

I LOST ALL FOUR GRANDPARENTS at an age when I was too young to appreciate their qualities or have a chance to talk to them to better understand my heritage and history. One of my grandmothers died at home in India after a long period of frailty from which she never recovered. She didn't have a terminal illness but a fall in old age followed by a badly fractured hip was enough to push her towards terminal decline. She developed a pressure ulcer and became confused and delirious, and in those days of very basic medicine, especially where we lived in India, her family could do little more except sit by her and soothe her through our presence. When she died, the rambling house fell literally quiet in the absence of her tortured screaming. But in its place descended a deep sadness and much soul-searching about how we could possibly have made her death better. Did we reveal our frustrations too often at her nocturnal whims? How many times did we hush her even when she didn't know what she was shouting? Did we accidentally ignore her pain, hunger or thirst?

Custom expected us to love and respect all our elders. My adolescent cousin devoted herself to our grandmother's skincare and hygiene with the skill and deft touch of a trained nurse, able to distinguish a cry of pain from a sob of gratitude. My grandmother's two sons did everything in their power to keep her well and sought out whatever medical care was available. But it was evident that she suffered at the end of life and it was a relief to us all when that suffering ended. As the last rites were fulfilled according to Hindu tradition and she lay on the funeral pyre, we hoped that she would join her husband in whatever lay beyond.

After the funeral, the house echoed with silence. We missed her so much that we had someone attend the house to summon her spirit from the afterlife, so we could communicate with her. It sounds slightly ridiculous now, but I remember how comforting it was to hear that she was okay. Humans will cling to any hope, however feeble.

My other grandmother succumbed to cancer. She died in a prominent Indian hospital, suspecting, but unaware to the end, that she had a terminal illness. She experienced none of the feared symptoms like pain, breathlessness or confusion, but she grew weaker by the day. In line with the times, her diagnosis was not disclosed to her and no one asked what she wanted at the end of life. To this day, in many cultures, it's unheard of to mention such things.

My grandmother was a devout woman who had begun each day by walking barefoot in a fasting state to pray at an ancient Hindu temple for god to keep her family safe. It is here she went to pray when one of her children got married, when a grandchild was born, and when someone fell ill. But before she went, she had to be satisfied that her large family was fed, which meant fanning a homemade fire, and later a rickety stove, since dawn. Sometimes, it would be nearly lunchtime by the time she set off to pray. A basket of flowers and beads in hand, she'd dash to the temple before it closed and hurry back, often ravenous but always fulfilled. One didn't have to agree with her philosophy, but it was impossible not to be moved by her discipline. For a long time after she died, people blamed her prolonged fasting habit for the cancer, but no one could say.

I can't help thinking that perhaps, if we had asked, she might have expressed a wish to go back home and spend her last days in the shadow of the same temple that had anchored her life. She would almost certainly have wanted to spend more time with her husband, children and grandchildren, and go home to sort out her few but carefully stored belongings. Instead, thinking we were helping, we urged her to stay in the best hospital in town for all her remaining days, so that doctors and nurses would fuss over her, giving her medicines that achieved nothing, while we waited for her to die.

One late night, we stole her away from under the eyes of the nurses to bless the vows of her youngest son, whose wedding had been hastily brought forward. The nurses were rightly mad when they found her missing from her bed and the oncologist didn't mince his words either. We were a little taken aback by their reaction and profusely apologetic but many years later, when I became an oncologist, it struck me that we only behaved like that because we knew that no doctor would dream of letting her out, leaving us feeling desperate. We regarded the professionals as omnipotent and omniscient but since we didn't know how to articulate our questions and they didn't think to broach difficult conversations, we fumbled in the dark, literally and metaphorically. All this sounds terrible in hindsight, but I know that this was the norm at the time and my grandmother received much better care than most.

As her liver failed, she slipped into a coma and died. In contrast to my other grandmother, who'd fractured her hip, her end from cancer was much more peaceful and controlled. She received good personal care and died with dignity but, astonishingly, the ripple impact of that death continues to

Dr Ranjana Srivastava

affect our family to this day. No one could have predicted that the tensions accumulated during that difficult period would create a rift among the siblings, their children and grandchildren that would lead to enduring pain and difficult questions decades later.

The family would be tasked with questions, not about whether her symptoms were managed (she didn't have many) or whether her death was preventable (it was not), but whether some frank conversations might have elicited her wishes about how she wanted to be remembered and who she wanted to leave her possessions to. Might her own expressed wishes have made a difference to those left behind? We will never know.

I offer these two personal memories to illustrate that no matter how ideal or imperfect a death, all survivors contend with some form of grief. In dealing with the gradual deterioration before death typical of the modern era, our mourning begins when people lose the qualities we best knew them for. Anticipating their death and letting go of our dreams for their future feels right and wrong in the same breath.

One of the privileges of my work is being allowed a window into how people cope with the aftermath of death.

Caring for the dying is all-consuming. Many family members throw themselves into this task with a kind of focus, abandon and passion that they may never have shown for anything else, even surprising themselves. This work is physically exhausting and emotionally challenging, so it's only natural that the finality of death creates a large hole and fuels many regrets. Relief from some of the physical aspects of caring is accompanied by many questions. Did we do enough? Did we say the right things? Could we have been better?

But the aftermath ought to be a time to console ourselves that we did what we could at the time. There are many ideas in human relationships that are not spelt out as well as we'd like, but we were there, we tried our best, and now we can rest easily. To be human is to be fallible.

One of the most painful things about the aftermath of death can be the doubts that surface in our head from time to time. It feels right to mourn the dead and only speak well of them since they are not there to defend themselves, but a corner of our mind can't help remembering how strained our relationship was and how angry, defensive or uncharitable they could be, even though we gave up some of the best years of our life being their friend, their carer, or both. I knew how conflicted I felt when a colleague said something unnecessarily harsh about a deceased friend we had both liked. To recollect his faults behind his back felt disloyal but to deny they ever existed was untrue. I understood then that even someone we loved and missed could be imperfect and acknowledging this didn't amount to denigrating the whole person.

Dr Ranjana Srivastava

I lost a late-term twin pregnancy days before I was to begin my first job as a specialist. The loss was as sudden as it was inexplicable and for months afterwards, eyeing the bump under my clothes, my patients would innocently ask when the baby was due. Of course, there was no baby and at the time, I feared if there would ever be one. The innocent anticipation of my patients would leave me outraged at the injustice of life and the unfairness of death – until I looked around me and realised that I was part of some grand scheme of life, magnificent and muddled at the same time. Some days, I wanted to lean into my grief, other days I wanted to run away as far as I could. One of the most poignant things to happen to me was an elderly patient telling me to take my time with grief. He had lost his wife of fifty years and everyone was impatient for him to move on, but he was quite happy to live beside her memory. My patient told me that the acute, raw, all-encompassing grief was too exhausting to sustain and would eventually dissipate, leaving in its place a dull ache that would flare without notice from time to time as a reminder that death never completely lost its hold. Time proved him correct. Since then, countless patients have taught me that all grief is legitimate and there is no hurry to vanquish it according to a timeline imposed by ourselves or another.

Society gives us greater permission to mourn a dead pet or a lost job than a loved one. We feel reluctant mentioning the dead, fearing that our words might visit bad luck or pour grief on the bereaved. We know how to celebrate an impending birth and mark the milestones of life, but we struggle to handle that other major event that must surely follow birth: death.

We mustn't hurry our sorrow merely to accommodate a world that's uncomfortable with the idea of mourning. Grief has no arc and bereavement doesn't follow a protocol. In an increasingly secular world, we may no longer adhere to the religion or customs of our ancestors, but we can still seek to be illuminated and consoled by how other people mourn.

Hindus cremate their dead as soon as possible and hold no rituals or prayers in their home for the next thirteen days as they await the departure of the soul, which they hold immortal, from the body. The one-month anniversary and the annual anniversary of the death are marked by special rites thought to bring peace to the dead and the living. Having taken part in these events, I have experienced the inner peace and closure they bring.

At the first notice of death, Muslims are taught to utter a verse from the Quran, 'To Allah we belong and truly, to Him we shall return.' The dead are usually buried within twenty-four hours after being washed and shrouded in modest cloth without seams or stitches. They are remembered through a special prayer where the congregation remains standing, but there are no formal ceremonies held after the funeral.

Buddhists believe the body is merely a vessel for the mind, which never ceases to exist. For up to a month after death, the body may exist in an intermediate state between birth and death and prayers during this time are open to everyone, including the recently bereaved and those who may be caring for the dying. The prayers are not to an entity, rather they're meant to produce clarity and purity of the mind.

Judaism also calls for an early burial of the deceased, following which Jews enter a period of deep mourning. For seven days after a person's death, they sit *shiva*, the Hebrew word for seven. Mourners sit low on the ground and share stories of the dead, wearing clothes that have been torn to symbolise a person torn from their lives. Friends and colleagues may visit at designated times to make a *shiva* call.

Christians have a strong belief in the afterlife and their funerals focus on the entry of the deceased into heaven. Hymns and prayers are offered for the soul of the deceased, hoping for their reawakening or believing that they have transcended into another life.

Some cultures mourn in private, while others require grief to be ostentatious in order to placate the deceased.

In contrast to the restraint shown in European cultures, the Congolese deem it shameful for a relative not to cry loudly at a funeral.

We can't say if the deceased are comforted, saddened or unmoved by the actions of those left behind but it's enough that we perform them to comfort us and grant us peace and reconciliation. The dead don't resent us for being alive nor do they wish us to grieve any more than we have. The dead are finally at rest – they'd be happy for us if our rituals helped us arrive at a place of peace.

Every Christmas, my family remembers this as we feel our grief anew. My husband's sister died unexpectedly at a young age and there was no time to say goodbye. The dinner table is not the same without her. Instead of setting a plate, we light a candle in her remembrance. Amidst the joy and bustle of Christmas, the flickering flame always evinces tears, but through this small but important gesture, we acknowledge our permanent sadness and teach our children that grief does not have an expiration date.

At a time when the consolations of religion have waned, there is a growing emphasis on seeking professional help during bereavement. This can help us navigate the worst parts of the grieving process, but I have learnt from the accounts of many patients that the passage of time and the togetherness of family are often the best healers.

Dr Ranjana Srivastava

Not everyone needs grief counselling – it's possible to hurt and recover on one's own. Upon the loss of my twin pregnancy, I was inundated with well-wishers and offers of help but all I needed was some time alone. Time, tears, quiet walks and writing all helped me right my topsy-turvy world. If they hadn't, I hope I'd have had the insight to seek help – sometimes, the value of professional help lies in reassuring us that our experience is normal.

When I meet relatives of my deceased patients, I always ask how they're coping. I'm reassured to hear that they have discovered themselves to be more resilient than they ever imagined, which speaks to the human capacity to endure and to recover. They tell me that their lives have been eased by making a new friend, finding fresh love, adopting a pet or trying a new hobby. Many emphasise the value of a routine in the aftermath of grief. This includes getting enough sleep, regular exercise, gentle socialisation and timely meals. One of the kindest gestures towards the bereaved is to be there for them as they face the future.

I always tell surviving relatives to return with their questions and concerns, knowing that this is one way of addressing the myths that occupy the minds of the bereaved long after everyone else has moved on. Every year, a handful of people accept the invitation and their stories are a poignant reminder of the regrets and fears that can accompany us in the aftermath of death. Other people turn to a longstanding family doctor, a social worker or palliative care professionals to make sense of their loss. Knowing that such thoughts are natural and common might empower us to ask questions long after we might think it irrelevant or impolite.

Almost no one experiences the death of a loved one without coming face to face with the subject of one's own mortality. We cannot be a close confidant, a constant carer or an involved friend at death without investing a large part of ourselves, hence it's only natural for death to prompt questions about our own destiny.

We need not be overwhelmed by them, but we cannot afford to banish them either. Rather, we would do well to invite an abundance of thoughts and ideas about dying as essential to a meaningful life. By reminding ourselves that we are mortal, we are treating ourselves with respect and being thoughtful towards those who will survive us.

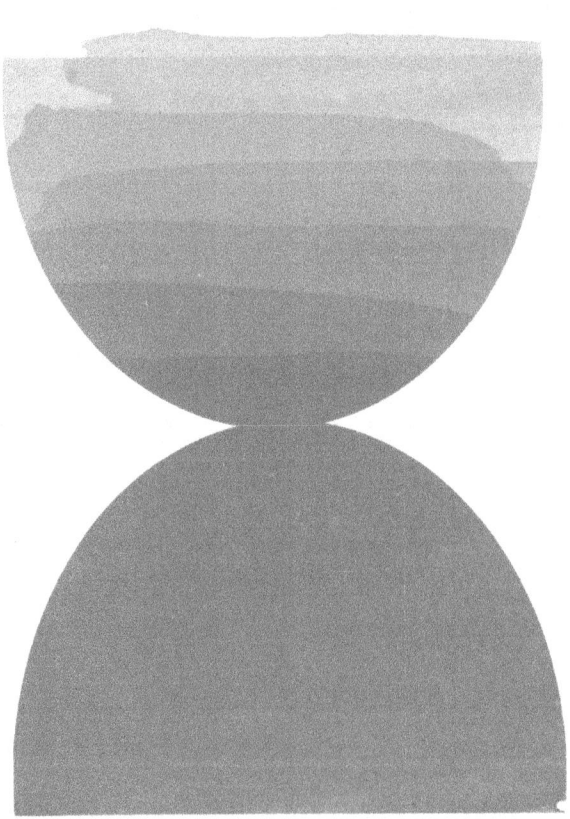

Epilogue

One of the hardest parts of being a doctor, in particular an oncologist, is to constantly run up against mortality. Death spares no one – neither the frail and elderly grandfather nor the beautiful and vibrant mother; neither the accomplished, urbane executive nor the hardworking, humble factory hand. Death is indeed the ultimate levelling experience. But instead of being limiting, this realisation has taught me to live each day meaningfully – to be grateful, mindful and useful. It's important to accept our mortality and live peacefully with it. The certainty of dying shouldn't dissuade us from living a full life and doing all we can to ensure it is healthy and long.

It is impossible to do my job without contemplating my legacy and reminding myself of the role I have in actively shaping it, whether it involves mentoring doctors, helping patients, or being a caring mother and a loyal friend. Most of all, it consists of being true to myself.

Even for someone who routinely cares for the dying, it is testing to imagine my own footprint erased from the world. I regard the fate of my young patients with heartache and dread, wondering how their children will cope. I am sobered by the loss of my oldest patients, especially when they still held an infectious enthusiasm for life. If I had a magic wand for a day, I think I might use it to erase loss that crops up in more ways than I can count.

It's striking how much death feels like a rebuke to modern medicine – a personal or professional failure rather than an assured thing. And I know all too well how easy it is to dismiss death as something that happens to others – in this, we are all given to magical thinking. But it's okay to be a work in progress. Indeed, we are all works in progress, coming to terms with the death of a loved one, contemplating our own mortality.

For most of us, death will come by way of a visible and gradual decline that's unlikely to be capped by going to sleep and never waking up. Our dying will involve months, sometimes years, of fluctuating health and a few near-misses.

There will be visits to emergency, close calls in intensive care, and an overwhelming parade of doctors interested in a part of us. Therefore, it will really fall to us to regard ourselves as more than the sum of our parts, as complex and unique individuals with dreams and desires and goals that matter. In order to honour them, we will need to actively shape our lives, knowing that a life well-lived is a stepping stone to a better death. How we do this is up to us, but the aim must be to keep at it.

I want to thank you for accompanying me on a difficult but important journey. I hope that some stories have inspired you, while others prompted you to think about who you are and where you are going. These are questions that face each and every one of us – we can answer them by being true to ourselves and by making space in our noisy and overexposed world for periods of silence and introspection.

Here's to your peace and fulfilment as you explore the makings of a good life and, ultimately, a better death.

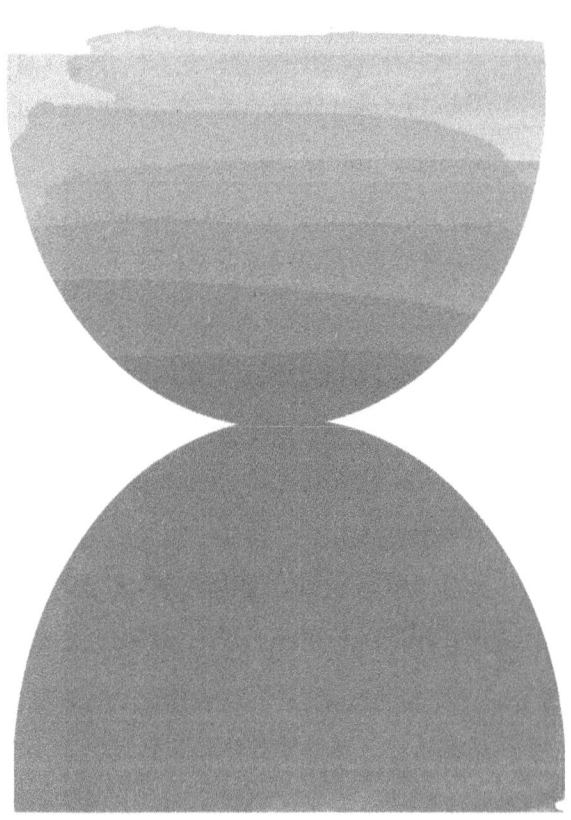

Acknowledgements

I START BY REPRISING MY DEDICATION. This book would not have been possible without the generosity of countless patients and their families, who have allowed me to care for them and shared their stories so that we may all learn from their experiences. To navigate one of life's most challenging events, the process of dying, and still retain the capacity and the will to care about others is extraordinary and I owe these selfless people a mountain of debt. They teach me how to be a better doctor and a more thoughtful person and I am confident that their stories will illuminate the lives of others.

Any creative process begins with someone believing in a vague idea. I thank my agent, Clare Forster, for reconnecting me with the wonderful Dan Ruffino of Simon & Schuster Australia, who could have said maybe, but chose to say yes and quietly empowered me to write this book. Claire de Medici, Katie Stackhouse, Shannon Kelly, Mark Evans and Lisa White have painstakingly transformed a disbanded draft into a real book, which always seems impossible until it isn't. The lovely Anna O'Grady and the sales team deserve praise for working tirelessly behind the scenes. As do Chris Lemoh, Irene Wagner, Kate Richards and Andrea McNamara and the team at *The Guardian* for helping me see further.

I reserve my greatest thanks for my publisher, Roberta Ivers, for two things – her diligent attention to my writing and her steadfast confidence in me. One cannot contemplate the weighty issue of what it means to live and die well without feeling uncertain and, sometimes, hopelessly lost. The task of an able publisher might be to simply redirect an author, but I've been enriched by Roberta's decency and friendship.

It's amazing that the love and support of my family has stayed constant through the demands of writing another book. For this, I thank my wonderful parents, Urmila and Kaushal, and my brother, Rajesh, for believing in me. I also thank Rosemary, Geoff, Taru and Helen for their support.

I would be a lesser writer without my husband, Declan, who specialises in conjuring ideas when he can't sleep and jotting them down for me while I sleep. To Rohan, Anjali and Sachin, thank you for your help in big and small ways. I'm lucky to have you and you know that there is no greater joy in my life than being your mother.

Ranjana Srivastava

About the Author

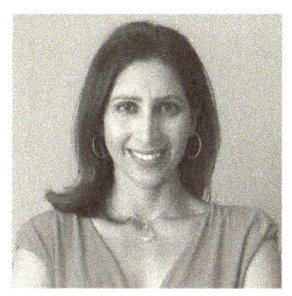

Dr Ranjana Srivastava OAM is a practising oncologist, internationally published and award-winning author, broadcaster and Fulbright scholar.

She is a fellow of the Royal Australasian College of Physicians and works in the public hospital system. In 2017, Ranjana was awarded the Medal of the Order of Australia for her contribution to doctor–patient communication and was recognised by Monash University as a Distinguished Alumni of the Year.

Her writing has been published worldwide, including in *Time* magazine and *The Week*, and in prominent medical journals such as *The New England Journal of Medicine*, *Lancet*, and *Journal of the American Medical Association*. In 2018 she was a finalist in the Walkley Awards for her work as a regular columnist for *The Guardian* newspaper. Her acclaimed non-fiction books include *Tell Me the Truth: Conversations with My Patients about Life and Death* (shortlisted, NSW Premier's Literary Awards), *Dying for a Chat: The Communication Breakdown Between Doctors and Patients* (winner, Human Rights Literature Prize) and *What It Takes to Be a Doctor* (finalist, Australian Career Book Award). She lives in Victoria.

See www.ranjanasrivastava.com